From Viral To Virile

The Fountain of Youth Isn't Just Real...It's Reachable

Praise for John Cisna

Creator of the *McDonald's Project*

"John's clarion call is more important now than when he first shocked the world just a few short years ago."

—Neil Cavuto, *Fox News*

"John Cisna has been in the public consciousness for a few years now, and this new book brings his story full circle. You'll learn everything that happened after his McDonald's experiment went viral, and discover the secrets of his new diet and exercise plan. We keep rooting for John and his bold exploits because he's one of us!"

—Zachary Hall, Author of *Don't Sleep On Planes*

"John has done what very few ever do—commit to a simple program that will change your life. Most people start a food and exercise program but fail to stay with it, in part, because it's not a sustainable program. John shows how easy and effective this program is without killing yourself at the gym or in the kitchen. Do yourself a favor—follow John's example laid out in this simple and easy-to-follow book."

—Brian Gaumer, Owner of *MuscleBoundUSA Gym*

"Every middle-aged person and older should read this book. Cisna takes health and wellness to another level. He describes his Fountain of Youth with such passion and energy that it makes you think, "I can do this!" His message of strength equals youth is spot on, and he delivers it with such simplicity it makes it believable and attainable."

—Mike Morsch, Author of *The Vinyl Dialogues* series

"Once again, John is blazing the trail for a better life with diet, exercise, and attitude. He creates a roadmap to a happier and healthier life for all of us. An entertaining read with stories and science throughout. John's enthusiasm and positive attitude is contagious!"

—Terry Garland, President/CEO, Garland and Associates

"John Cisna has a way of bringing everything to your level (no matter what that might be) in a very common sense manner. And now he's at it again, educating us on a way to get stronger and live longer, with himself as the guinea pig. As with his original McDonald's Project, John has the empirical data to substantiate his results and quantify his findings. It's a terrific, inspiring story!"

—Mike George

"I had the pleasure of coaching John Cisna and watched him distinguish himself as an All-State baseball player. John has always looked for new and better ways to present his ideas, so a book about fitness is no surprise to me. He's put a great deal of time, research, and his own experience into this book. Many people could and should benefit from it."

—Jim Mahoney, Retired Teacher/Coach, Johnston High School

"This book really brings home the point about life and the choices one makes about diet, exercise, health issues, learning curves, individual body differences, and commitment. You gave me a lot to think about!"

—Sharon Montgomery

"You can just feel John Cisna's enthusiasm—I immediately decided to incorporate the diet into my daily life. It's so exciting to think that working out and eating right doesn't have to be complicated."

—Ellen Feller

"This is the most important book for weight loss. It shows that eating less is not a good solution, because it slows down your metabolism. Instead, the Cisna lifestyle helps you lose weight permanently by improving your hormones. Highly recommended for patients and professionals."

—Dr. Salomon Jakubowicz, Endocrinology

"I've learned many valuable lessons from John Cisna about the importance of my decisions, whether in my life, in the classroom, or on the golf course. This book opens my eyes towards the choices I make concerning my health. I'm young and healthy, and I want to stay that way for a long time. Everything happens for a reason and I like to be in charge of those reasons."

—Zoee Risdal, former student

From Viral To Virile

The Fountain of Youth Isn't Just Real...It's Reachable

John Cisna

With Ed Sweet

John Cisna is available for speaking engagements.
To make arrangements, please write to info@johncisna.net

First print edition ISBN: 978-1-62249-418-7
First e-book edition/eISBN: 978-1-62249-423-1

Cover Photograph by Tom Wagner
Cover Design by Pam Barton
Interior Design by Terrie Scott

10 9 8 7 6 5 4 3 2 1

Note to Readers
This book is sold with the understanding that the authors and publisher are not rendering medical advice of any kind. This book is not intended to replace medical advice, or to diagnose, prescribe, or treat any disease, condition, illness, or injury. Before you begin any diet or exercise program, receive full medical clearance from a licensed physician. The authors and publisher of this book claim no responsibility to any person or entity for any liability, loss, or damage caused or alleged to be caused, directly or indirectly, as a result of the use, application, or interpretation of the material contained herein.

This book is dedicated to the countless individuals who've struggled with finding their path to health. My hope is that this book will turn the light on in the attic for anyone who wants to experience the same "wow" factor that I have in discovering what really works. The Fountain of Youth is real, and, more importantly, it's attainable for everyone.

This book explains how I found that fountain and how you can too. I truly believe that living life to its fullest is a combination of the right food plan and being physically strong. Go get it—it's out there for you!

—John Cisna

Table of Contents

Foreword

Fat Chance the Food Police Will Ever Admit
John Cisna Was Right, Even Now

His story is now legendary. In a span of little more than six months, John Cisna lost 54 pounds, eating at McDonald's. Yeah, McDonald's. He thinned down going to the same place Morgan Spurlock famously pigged out. Spurlock got a hit movie out of it, *Super Size Me*, and with a single stroke of his fork, and more often a lot of paper wrappers, managed to alienate not only McDonald's but the entire fast food industry.

Back to John, who seemed to conclude maybe Spurlock was eating all the wrong stuff, or too much of the wrong stuff. The difference was, of course, Spurlock's story fed a media narrative that fast food was bad, and McDonald's was the worst. Cisna's story didn't make sense, so it didn't garner nearly as much coverage.

It's a pity because Cisna proved something that should be so common sense, it needn't take a hit documentary to pound over your head—it's not what you eat, it's how much of what you eat that matters. French fries aren't evil. Maybe downing a couple of super-size servings of them every day is.

That was Cisna's agenda then, when he lost all that weight. That's his agenda now, as he miraculously maintains that weight and all the good health that comes with it. As he puts it, "I was perfectly happy overeating at fine restaurants and binging on food obtained at the grocery store. Trust me, if you eat too much of any food, I can guarantee you that you'll eventually become obese."

McDonald's proved his challenge because making McDonald's a target for all our health ills has become pretty much the media diet. Besides exploring personal responsibility, John this time gets into something else—personal freedom.

John Cisna

"Not everything on the McDonald's menu is filled with salt and fat," John writes now. In fact, he's included the fast food giant in a common sense list of eating venues, recognizing the obvious. "Fast food is here to stay," he concludes.

For one thing, it's easy. For another, it's fast. And in our time-crunched society that's a fairly compelling business model that has and will continue to stand the test of time.

But what John reveals here is that the easy and fast choice needn't be bad and dangerous. Far from it. Common sense choices that customers make, and not the choices the fast food police make, dictate how our bodies hold up and whether our weight stays down.

That's why John's clarion call is more important now than when he first shocked the world just a few short years ago. Take it from his success and his still trim figure. But more, take it from me. Back in 2016, I had open-heart surgery, a hastily arranged triple-bypass for which I wasn't prepared and my common sense approach to food wasn't anywhere near John's.

I learned the hard way. Bad choices yield bad results. Good choices yield good results. Leave it to John to figure that out without having to have his chest ripped open. Word to the wise—don't pay short shrift to a guy who's laying out surviving for the long haul.

It's what we eat, yes. But more, it's how we live. John taught a nation discussing the former. He brings it to a whole new level now, expounding on the latter. I like to call it a blueprint for never being blue, for never letting weight or bad choices bog you down. Through diet, exercise, and just everyday common sense guidelines, John reminds us that it's up to US.

Spurlock's agenda was to target McDonald's. I think John's agenda is to target us. He wants us to quit making excuses, and start making choices. We control our fate—whether it's staring at a filled fork or an unused treadmill.

It's about persistence, but more, as John reveals here in this very handy guide to living right, it's about being patient. Sadly, there are no short-term fixes. Thinking there are puts us in only a bigger fix. The only thing John is super-sizing here is practical advice—in heaping servings.

McDonald's isn't his target. We are. We all are. He's not here to point fingers. He is here to point us all in the right direction. Without the cheap shots—without any shots. He's real. His advice is sincere, and his mission undeniable. It's reflected in the pastor-like zeal he brings to his purpose—not to have us answer to our better angels but simply, better health. Not bad, not bad at all.

Maybe because he's not angry or placing blame, John brings the fat and thin alike on a path toward "body peace." You can do that when you've done that. John's done that. John lives that. Look at him. Read him. Understand him. Imitate him. What have you got to lose, but some pounds and maybe some clogged arteries.

Take it from a remarkable lifestyle evangelist who practices the healthy lifestyle he preaches. But also take it from me, someone decidedly not, who's here to tell you it's never too late to say you still might have a prayer...just yet.

Neil Cavuto
Anchor, Managing Editor and Sr. Vice President
Fox News Channel
Fox Business Network

Introduction

No one can tell me that I don't have balls. At age fifty-four, I turned a high school science experiment into a viral media sensation that resulted in a two-and-a-half-year contract with one of the world's largest franchisors, McDonald's. I endured jealousy from friends and colleagues who resented my fifteen minutes of fame, and I was the target of an aggressive "food advocate" whose petition against my presentation for McDonald's led to a barrage of social media attacks that had me fearing for my safety.

While I had the cajones to weather the whirlwind that was my life from January 2014 through December 2016, what I didn't know was that my testosterone levels were on the low end of normal. Like most middle-aged men, my body's supply of this essential hormone probably began decreasing in my thirties, bringing me to about half of what I had when I was in the prime of my life.

I was on an emotional high with the success of my McDonald's experiment, but I didn't know about the physical low that plagued me at the same time. I've since come to realize how dangerous having low levels of testosterone can be, for both men and women.

For guys, low testosterone doesn't just lead to a low libido. Insufficient testosterone is one of the major contributing factors to the deadly belly fat that often accumulates as we get older. We don't get those spare tires just from overeating! Low T can also result in poor cognitive function, and has been linked to serious conditions like type 2 diabetes, cardiovascular disease, and prostate cancer. As you'll learn later in this book, a shortage of testosterone in men makes death—from ANY cause—much more likely.

Women need testosterone, too, and while they don't need a lot of it, it needs to be in the right balance to keep their bones healthy, manage pain, preserve cognitive function, and even increase sex drive after menopause.

The Pinnacle of Health Is Possible

After my experience with McDonald's ran its course, I began to think about what I could do to really make myself healthier. If I could lose 54 pounds eating nothing but McDonald's for six months, imagine what I could do if I looked for a food program specifically designed for my individual physiology to maximize health and combined it with a great exercise program!

One of the most important lessons I learned from my McDonald's experiment was that it felt a whole lot better to weigh 226 pounds than it did to weigh 280. So, after my commitment to the Golden Arches came to an end, I decided to try to make myself as healthy and as strong as I could possibly become.

This new experiment has been so wildly successful for me that I just had to share the news. So now I'm on a mission to reach as many people as possible with the message that the Fountain of Youth is real. Anyone who can't see how a few simple choices are game changers when it comes to health and vitality has got to be a few fries short of a Happy Meal!

I know that eating right and exercising isn't easy, but I'm here to tell you about a training regimen that fits into any schedule and a healthy diet that tastes good and lets you eat mass quantities of food.

At fifty-eight years old, I'm stronger, healthier, and happier than I've ever been in my life. I can deadlift 385 pounds. My romantic life with my wife of thirty-seven years is fifty shades of awesome. And, at a time when most guys my age are dreaming of a leisurely retirement, I'm working two jobs, writing books, speaking all over the country, and helping men and women just like me find practically unlimited energy by making better choices about exercise and nutrition.

I'm not here to brag about myself. I'm no different than anyone else. And if I can reach my own personal pinnacle of health, you can do it, too. While I'm proud of my accomplishments, the real reason I talk about them is to inspire people—specifically YOU, my friend—to take charge of their own lives and live them to the absolute fullest.

Strength by Numbers

I've always loved science, because data doesn't lie. The reason my McDonald's project went viral is because the results were real and went beyond my obvious and significant weight loss. In addition to the 54 pounds I lost, my ongoing blood work through the course of the experiment kept moving in the right direction.

Ninety days into the experiment my total cholesterol was down 32 percent, my triglycerides were down by 49 percent, my LDL was down 34 percent, and my cholesterol-to-HDL ratio dropped by 20 percent.

My current health and fitness experiment is also data driven. You'll not only see the results of my blood work, but I'll also impress you with some phenomenal strength gains achieved by a middle-aged guy who never lifted a weight before. Just take a quick look at how much I improved in four months in the core exercises that make up my new program:

- Military Press—130% strength increase
- Bent Over Row—150% strength increase
- Bench Press—153% strength increase
- Deadlift—170% strength increase
- Squat—182% strength increase

While the raw data is compelling in and of itself, it's really the real-life impact that provides the true meaning behind an experiment like this. In my current journey, I've met lots of people who've used the techniques I've been applying to my own life to better themselves physically, emotionally, and spiritually.

How Far Can You Take Yourself?

As human beings, we have the potential to use better health to improve so many important aspects of our lives. In this book, I'm going to share some powerful stories from my own life, and the lives of others, to show you what's possible and inspire you to achieve great things. I'm driven to find answers to many of the problems men and women face at any age, particularly as we get older. You know, things like these:

- How can we feel relevant in the career world?
- How can we rekindle romance?
- How can we win at the wonderful game of life?
- How can we maximize our time spent exercising?
- How can we eat for optimal health?
- How can we deal with the haters in the world?
- How can we handle fame and notoriety?

In addition to being a story about my journey toward ultimate healthfulness, this book is also a commentary on the media machine that tells us what's cool, what's good, what's inappropriate, and what's controversial.

I'll take you through the highs and lows of the years I spent as a McDonald's brand ambassador. You'll learn why I was kicked out of schools, why franchise owners are among the best people on the planet, and how a company can try too hard to craft the "right" message.

And with no more connections to McDonald's, or any other entity, I'm going to explain some of the secrets I've learned about losing weight, gaining muscle, increasing testosterone, becoming stronger, and never being afraid to take a chance in life.

I'm living proof that you're never too old to reinvent yourself or take on new challenges that can lead to incredible personal growth. It all comes down to making informed choices that fit your age, condition, and lifestyle, and committing to those choices because the rewards of making them are so great.

Tap Into the Power of Choice

This idea of choice was often lost on people who heard about my McDonald's experience. Certain individuals were so conditioned to believe that fast food was bad that they couldn't see the simplicity of my experiment. Basically, all I was saying was that if you limit your calories to around 2,000 a day—after years of eating between 4,000 and 5,000 calories a day—you're going to lose weight.

McDonald's was just the attention-getting vehicle for this very mundane and logical fact. Indeed, it was the unique context of my particular experiment that definitely put people in two opposing camps. For McDonald's supporters, especially the network of owner/operators around the world, I was a godsend. Finally, they had a counter argument against Morgan Spurlock's popular 2004 documentary *Super Size Me*.

But for people who hated McDonald's specifically, and fast food in general, I was the Antichrist. People who never met me or took the time to investigate what I was really saying launched a campaign that would eventually prevent me from speaking to kids in middle and high schools, despite the fact that the hundreds of teachers and thousands of students who had already seen me speak not only got my message of balance and personal accountability, but also gave me high marks for it.

Despite all the naysayers, my message is basically the same as it's always been—that the choices we make in life largely determine our outcomes.

If you can understand this, then you're way ahead of a lot of people. But don't let the simplicity of this message fool you. If you can make good choices with intention, and if you can keep doing so, you can make powerful changes in your life.

You're making a choice right now to read this book, and hopefully it will lead to a good outcome for you. You can choose to follow my program in a quest to become healthier, or you can choose some other program that works for you. You can even choose to think I'm an idiot and throw the book away, but I really hope you don't do that.

Maybe the choices you make will work for you, maybe they won't. But even choices that don't get you the results you want can be teachable moments. That's why I love data and rely on it so much. If my blood work goes bad, or if my strength gains disappear, I can make new choices in the form of adjustments. These might be small or they might be large, but I always have an opportunity to correct course.

John Cisna

Join Me on the Path to a Stronger, Healthier, More Youthful You

Regardless of what you choose to do, I hope I can inspire you to make good choices when it comes to living your best, loving your best, eating your best, and functioning at your best in a strong, healthy body.

I've discovered an exercise program and a food plan that have helped me gain energy and vitality, as well as lean muscle and increased testosterone. This is a total program that's working wonders for me, and I encourage you to talk to your doctor to see if it's right for you, too.

I can't stress how important it is to have a doctor to consult. I've had the same doctor do my blood work since I started my McDonald's experiment in 2013. As you'll see in the pages that follow, he's been a great resource for me, as were numerous other doctor friends.

It's my sincere hope that you can find your own Fountain of Youth that you can drink from for the rest of your days. Whether you follow my program or find another one that works for you, I hope that I can leave you with the knowledge that only YOU are in charge of your destiny. Only YOU can make the choices that will bring you a better life. Only YOU can push your limits, rise above your critics, and forge the change you want in your world, whether it's a healthier body, a better love life, a more interesting career, or just the freedom to be yourself despite anything anyone else has to say about it.

Let's get started

Chapter One

I Proved That Fast Food Isn't Fat Food
But There Are Still People Who Don't Believe It!

Conventional wisdom is funny. Sometimes things that are accepted as true are factual, but sometimes they aren't.

Take fast food, for example. If you ask most people, they'd probably admit that it's not the healthiest food out there. The idea that fast food is bad for you has become conventional wisdom, and that made it easy for documentary filmmaker Morgan Spurlock to find great success with a 2004 movie called *Super Size Me*.

This admittedly compelling movie showed what people believed all along—that if you eat fast food, you're going to get obese, lose energy, feel like crap, and dramatically increase your risk of a heart attack, liver damage, and other life-threatening and expensive medical conditions.

What Morgan Spurlock did was provide evidence that fit conventional wisdom about fast food, and the creative way he did it really hurt McDonald's. Under pressure from the movie's message, the fast-food giant eliminated its supersize options just six weeks after the film's release and began adding healthier menu items at about the same time. More than ten years later when I came on the scene, the McDonald's owner/operators I encountered all told me that I was the answer to Morgan Spurlock they'd been looking for all that time!

Spurlock became the very public spokesperson for a long list of people who wanted to vilify the fast-food industry in general and McDonald's in particular. Passionate people really believed that McDonald's and other fast-food chains were responsible for America's obesity epidemic, and the fact that these heartless companies marketed food to kids made the whole industry's crimes that much more heinous.

John Cisna

Morgan Spurlock actually got the idea for his film while watching a news report about parents who were accusing McDonald's of making their two teen daughters obese. Never mind the fact that the report was actually about the judge dismissing the lawsuit!

Spurlock Had an Agenda, and So Did I

When *Super Size Me* hit the theaters—big purveyors of popcorn, candy, hot dogs, pretzels, and other unhealthy foods by the way—the war on McDonald's and fast food intensified. What people didn't seem to understand about the documentary, however, was that all the physical problems Morgan Spurlock developed over the course of his thirty-day McDonald's consumption were related to the choices he made, not to the food itself.

Spurlock's experiment was designed to paint McDonald's as the bad guy. He didn't follow the Food and Drug Administration (FDA) dietary guidelines for calories or for any of the key nutrients for which the government provides recommendations. Instead, he decided he would agree to eat more food whenever a McDonald's employee asked if he wanted to supersize his order. In a free society, no one has to answer yes to that question every time it's asked.

But Spurlock had an agenda, which is fine. He was fit and healthy to begin with, and it wouldn't have been much of a story if he stayed fit and healthy after eating McDonald's. For stories to be compelling, people have to undergo dramatic change. And Morgan Spurlock wanted his health to get worse.

So he ate more than he normally did. A lot more. And it made him throw up. It made him gain weight. And it affected his liver. *Super Size Me* didn't show me that fast food is bad—it showed me that if you make bad choices with fast food, you could damage your body.

I rarely ate fast food before my McDonald's experiment. In fact, I didn't need fast food to gain excess fat. I was perfectly happy overeating at fine restaurants and binging on food obtained at the grocery store. Trust me, if you eat too much of ANY food, I can guarantee that you'll eventually become obese.

When I did my McDonald's experiment, I also had an agenda. Not to say that McDonald's food was healthy, but to prove Morgan Spurlock wrong by making different choices with the same food. It's not the food that's bad, it's the choices we make with the food we have available that can hurt us. I'm not saying it's easy to make good choices, but it certainly is possible if you put your mind to it. What Morgan Spurlock and I both did was to show how different choices can lead to very different outcomes.

I Didn't Set Out to Be Controversial

I never dreamed there'd be so much controversy over the simple experiment I conducted. I just wanted to demonstrate, through empirical data, that it's possible to lose weight even if the only thing you eat is fast food.

To refresh your memory, from October 1, 2013, through March 31, 2014, I ate nothing but McDonald's for breakfast, lunch, and dinner and I lost 54 pounds—the equivalent of a small child. When I started the experiment, my stomach measured fifty-one inches around. To put that in perspective, that's pretty much the circumference of a hula hoop.

By the end of the six months, I had slimmed down to a waist size of forty inches and had to buy all new pants. It didn't happen because I was eating at McDonald's all the time. It happened because I was eating at McDonald's all the time and *limited* my calories to about 2,000 a day.

The McDonald's menu was simply my grocery store for half a year. And I had a lot more healthy options to choose from than Mr. Spurlock did ten years earlier. Egg White Delights and oatmeal were among my favorite breakfast choices. I had salads and Fruit 'N Yogurt Parfaits for lunch. But I wasn't shy about eating burgers and fries for dinner, and I sometimes treated myself to some ice cream. Everything was fair game as long as I stayed within my daily calorie count. In fact, I ate better at McDonald's for six months than I did for years before I started the experiment.

My outstanding weight loss and impressive blood work proved conclusively that food is not the cause of the obesity epidemic in this country. Yet critics of what I was doing just couldn't see the message. They were either blinded by conventional wisdom, or invested in destroying McDonald's for selling what they perceived as unhealthy food.

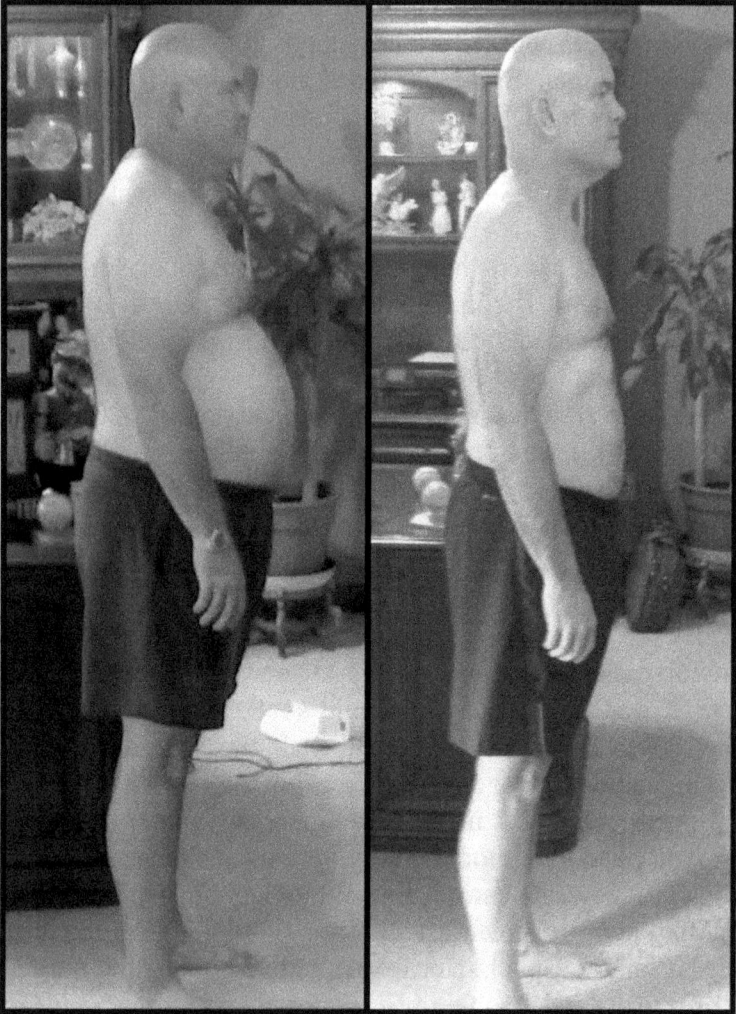

My before and after photos during my McDonald's experiment. I lost a total of 54 pounds eating nothing but McDonald's for six months.

Even before my experiment became a national media sensation, I should have seen the controversy coming. People at my school in Colo, Iowa, couldn't believe that I lost 54 pounds eating 540 meals at McDonald's. Even though I was shrinking before their very eyes, several of my colleagues—all smart, well-educated individuals—let their preconceived notions of fast food blind them to the truth of what I was doing.

The controversy escalated exponentially when my experiment made me famous. You might have seen my exchange with Joy Bauer, a health and nutrition expert and contributor on the *TODAY* show. On national television she berated me for consuming too much sodium during my McDonald's experiment. While my sodium intake was definitely something I couldn't keep within the FDA dietary guidelines, it seemed odd that she would focus on that so intently instead of on all the other positive aspects of the project. In fact, sodium was the only nutritional factor of the fifteen we tracked that fell outside the guidelines in a potentially negative way. Most of the other fourteen, including fat, cholesterol, fiber, calcium, and even sugar, were either within a few percentage points of the FDA number or were outside the range in a positive way.

Joy seemed like she had to find a way to reveal how evil it is for the fast-food industry to use sodium to preserve their food. I'm not sure if it's evil, but if it is, it's a necessary ingredient that comes along with processed food. In my individual case, the extra sodium wasn't really a factor because I'm not salt sensitive and I've always had perfect blood pressure.

And quite frankly, new research has come out about salt that suggests that the current dietary guidelines may not be correct. I refer you to a *New York Times* article from May 8, 2017, called "Why Everything We Know About Salt May Be Wrong," which explains how "new studies of Russian cosmonauts, held in isolation to simulate space travel, show that eating more salt made them *less* thirsty but somehow hungrier. Subsequent experiments found that mice burned more calories when they got more salt, eating 25 percent more just to maintain their weight."

I'm going off on a tangent here and I want to bring you back to my story and all the controversy it created. Things got really bad when I became a brand ambassador for McDonald's and started speaking at schools across the country. I'll explain more about this in the next chapter, but a self-described food advocate led an entire campaign to shut me down and prevent me from speaking at schools because she believed I was encouraging kids to not only eat fast food, but also consume mass quantities of McDonald's!

Before this person came after me, I had already spoken at about a hundred different schools. And I have to tell you that I never heard once from a teacher or student that they felt free to binge on fast food. It was quite the opposite. My message of choice and balance was the one that resonated, and that's why I repeatedly got standing ovations and positive feedback and letters from every audience I spoke to.

I totally understand that fair-minded people can disagree about the effects of fast-food marketing and the intentions of fast-food chains, but to claim that the only reason McDonald's does its charitable work, educational work, and anti-bullying outreach is to increase market share is the ultimate cynicism. I have no reason to doubt it when people claim to be concerned parents. But guess what? I'm also a concerned parent, and so are the thousands of people who own and work at McDonald's franchises.

Are You Smarter Than a Seventh Grader?

When I got back to Colo after my whirlwind media trip to New York, a student in my seventh grade life science class raised her hand to ask me a question. When I called on her, she said, "Mr. Cisna, we're having a hard time understanding all of this. Isn't all you and the sophomores did nothing more than common sense? Why is this such a big deal?"

She was so right. Why was this McDonald's experiment so big? All we did was follow government dietary guidelines, for goodness sake! I find it funny that seventh graders have it figured out but I would spend the next three years of my life trying to convince the rest of the world of the same thing.

I explained to this young lady, and to the class as a whole, that she was right. I said that many people spend too much time clinging to long-standing beliefs and refuse to be open to the fact that they might actually be wrong. The empirical data from my experiment really made it tough for people, because how can you argue, or rationalize, beliefs that don't coincide to the data?

Teachers Can Learn Lessons Too

I'm the first to admit that I'm a simple man who did a simple experiment to expose the fallacy of the conventional wisdom around fast food, and show people that they could lose weight by making better choices. I never once claimed that McDonald's food is nutritious or not nutritious. I never encouraged anyone to eat more fast food or less fast food. All I set out to do was show that our choices have a huge impact on every aspect of our lives.

In hindsight, I probably shouldn't have put my daily meals in the first book I wrote. It kind of gave the impression that I was advocating an all-fast-food diet plan, when all I really wanted to do by showing everything I ate was satisfy people's curiosity and the need for transparency. I was also hoping to point out that if you found yourself in a pinch, you could put together a diet of fast food for a day or two that wouldn't adversely affect your life. So I put every one of the meals, along with the corresponding caloric information, in the back of my book.

Even though I had a disclaimer in the book, McDonald's got nervous about it when we were in negotiations about how we might work together.

It was actually one of the first things that came up when we started talking. They wanted all publication stopped and any unsold inventory pulled.

The funny thing was that I wrote the book with their knowledge prior to our agreement, but they never provided any input because they didn't think I'd get it published in the time frame I told them we would. I told them I wanted to have the book done in seven weeks and they thought that was impossible. Large corporations move a lot slower than highly motivated individuals trying to capitalize on unexpected media attention, so, needless to say, they were shocked when I showed them the finished product and told them I had plans to publish it in paperback and electronic formats. The book was way down the road and there was no turning back.

I understood where they were coming from when they told me to pull the book, and it was the first inkling I got about the different set of rules and regulations that big companies like

McDonald's have to abide by. I found out very quickly that the Federal Trade Commission (FTC) enforces many regulations regarding diet claims, and evidently my book broke every one of them!

As an individual I was fine, but if I were connected with the corporation in any way, the book would have caused multiple legal headaches for McDonald's. This was just one of the many lessons I'd learn as I embarked on the new chapter of my life as a McDonald's brand ambassador, and I'll tell you about it all in the next chapter.

Healthy or Not? You Decide.

I still get asked quite often if I think McDonald's food is really healthy. My answer is simple. All foods have a "health" factor. The challenge for each one of us is to find out what foods will give us the right balance of nutrients, taste, pleasure, etc. If we make good choices overall, we can make room for some treats for healthy lives we fully enjoy. Even the strictest diets allow a little bit of cheating, and if that means you decide to go and get a Big Mac once in a while, is that really so bad?

Not everything on the McDonald's menu is filled with salt and fat. Many of the chain's egg dishes, salads, chicken sandwiches, snacks, etc., are perfectly acceptable choices, even when consumed on a regular basis. Joy Bauer and others don't have confidence that people who go to McDonald's can avoid the seductive power of the menu items with the worst nutritional value. They think everyone who walks into McDonald's becomes magically mesmerized by the sights and smells of crispy fries and juicy burgers. They might be tempting, but the decision to choose those particular menu items consistently can't be the exclusive fault of the fast-food chain

The one major point I tried to make with my McDonald's project is that we have to quit blaming fast food, or any other food, for our health issues. We all have many choices available to us. Nobody puts a gun to our heads and says, "Eat fast food or else!"

Do I continue to eat fast food today? Rarely, but on occasion I will.

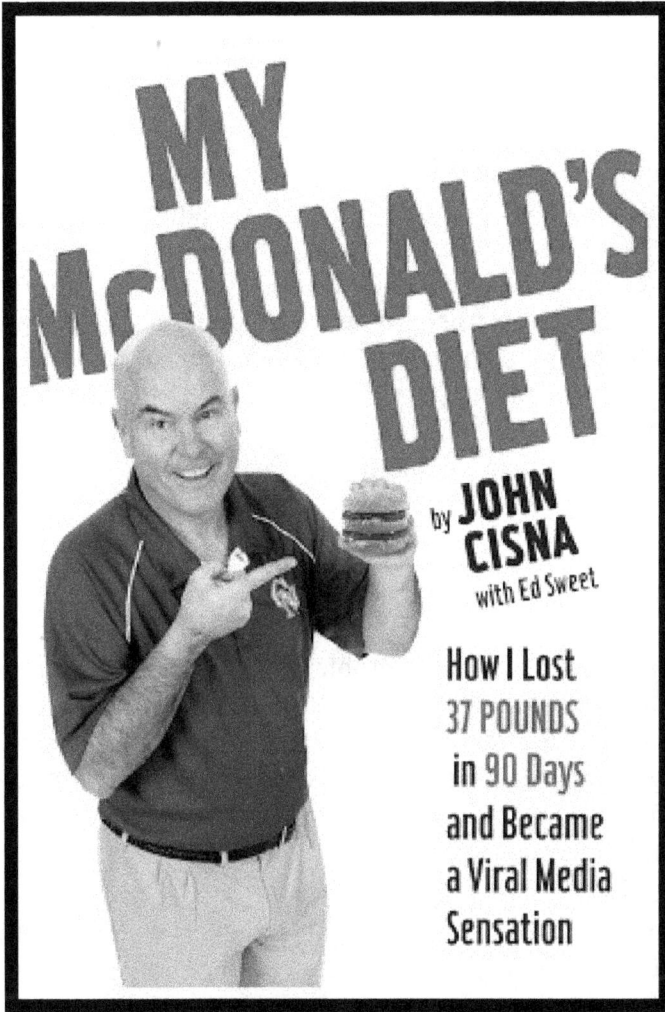

My first book was pulled from the shelves when
I started working as a McDonald's brand ambassador.

If I were on the road and had to eat fast food would I pull over and eat at McDonald's? Without question I would! I've been fortunate enough to be behind the scenes at Hamburger University and various food-processing plants. I marvel at the care that McDonald's takes to ensure their foods are 100 percent safe for consumption, and I know that the company's menu items have a level of nutrition that's more than adequate for me in short-term situations.

15

John Cisna

Fast food isn't part of my regular food plan today, but I have to credit McDonald's for getting me on the road to better health. I wouldn't be as healthy as I am now if it hadn't been for my McDonald's experiment and how it all unfolded with the media flurry and my experience as a brand ambassador.

My challenge to you is to start thinking about the choices you're making, and evaluate what you're doing to see if you've found a path to overall health and happiness. Are you heading toward the best you possible, or are you getting lost in the woods? If you need a little redirection, I'm here to give it to you in the form of a program that works not just for my personal physiology, but for a lot of people I've met on my new journey to becoming as healthy as I can possibly be as a unique human being with a specific genetic makeup.

Patience Is a Virtue

Part of our societal problem with weight control is that people want fast fixes rather than long-term success plans. Immediate gratification plays a huge role in people's decisions regarding weight loss. I've learned that whenever I see a plan advertised as losing "X" amount of weight quickly, I usually head for the hills, because short-term fixes do not set you up for long-term success.

My McDonald's experiment and the one I'm working on today have taught me that the key to successful weight loss is making a consistent commitment to real lifestyle change. Fortunately, I find it pretty easy to stick to something, and even Thanksgiving didn't deter me from eating McDonald's back in 2013.

If there's one paramount piece of information that I can pass on about sticking to a new lifestyle plan it's this: BE PATIENT! You've got to get over that quick-fix mentality, because if you don't, you'll just get anxious and give up when you don't get the results you want fast enough.

During my McDonald's project, I made the mistake of weighing myself every day. I really freaked out on those days when, despite sticking to my plan, I actually went up in weight by a pound or two. Those fluctuations are natural, and when I went back and looked at my weight on a week-by-week basis, all the data points showed consistent weight loss.

Another tip is to avoid being swayed by pictures of people in advertisements who are absolutely ripped with muscles. Those people are at the far right side of the bell curve when it comes to the genes that govern physical appearance. Most of us are AVERAGE people, so instead of competing with the naturally gifted, just compete with yourself and enjoy the improvements you make every day.

Remember, you have exactly the same number of muscles that Mr. Universe has. Do what it takes to make the most of them and you'll enjoy long-term success that intertwines nicely with your everyday lifestyle.

Fast Food Is Here to Stay

If we're being realistic about things, fast food won't be going away anytime soon. In fact, CNN recently released a study that shows how pervasive fast food is among every section of our society, from rich to poor.

The research revealed "the guilty pleasure of enjoying a McDonald's hamburger, Kentucky Fried Chicken popcorn nuggets, or Taco Bell burrito is shared across the income spectrum…with an overwhelming majority of every group reporting having indulged at least once over a nonconsecutive three-week period."

Our busy schedules make fast food the best solution at times, so I'm not surprised about the research at all. I'm not sure I'd call it a guilty pleasure, however, since sometimes it's not pleasurable at all and you're just in a hurry! For better or for worse, the genie is out of the bottle and fast food will ALWAYS be a part of everyday life. If people believe we could somehow snap our fingers and eliminate every fast-food restaurant on earth and thus eliminate obesity, they're seriously kidding themselves.

I honestly believe that even if fast food went away, our obesity problem would be much greater than it is today. My weight was out of control for most of my adult life and fast food was an extremely small part of my diet. I got fat from eating food from grocery stores and sit-down restaurants.

Using fast food as a scapegoat might be as convenient as eating at a fast-food restaurant, but it really doesn't get us anywhere. It all comes back to choice.

It took me six months of my life and 540 straight McDonald's meals to get on a path to health. The baseline I started at was pretty terrible. I weighed 280 pounds and had a cholesterol level of 249. My triglycerides were 156 and my LDL was 170.

All that is different now. Eating at McDonald's for six months inspired me to get even healthier, and that's why I'm sharing my experiences with you today.

So even though I know I'll never convince everybody, I hope you're one person who joins me in the belief that fast food isn't fat food.

Chapter Two

My Life as a Brand Ambassador

It's a safe bet to say that I'm one of the oldest people to go viral on the Internet. I was fifty-four years old when I flew to New York to tell my story on the *TODAY* show, *Fox & Friends*, and *Your World with Neil Cavuto*. And after forty-eight hours in the Big Apple, my life changed forever.

Words simply cannot describe how fast things were moving at that point for me. People I hadn't seen or talked to in years were all getting in touch to find out what it was like to be "famous." I was getting calls from every news outlet imaginable. Later on I would be asked to do product endorsements. It was absolutely out of control, and when I was in New York, I had to literally shut my phone off for several hours just to catch my breath and get my faculties back.

I thought about hiring a manager or a publicist to handle all the media requests and map out a strategy for how to take full advantage of my unique situation, but that's when I started hearing rumblings that McDonald's might see some value in having me work for them in some capacity.

All the publicity associated with my experiment definitely got the attention of the corporate giant. Many of the owner/operators I knew were trying to get me in the door, and they relayed to me that key people in the corporate offices thought I might be able to improve the company's image.

Frankly, McDonald's never had such a positive situation land in their laps like they did with my experiment, which was the third most viral story of 2014. My experiment was the first thing in ten years that McDonald's could point to, in a concrete and reputable way, to counter Morgan Spurlock and his twisted documentary *Super Size Me*. So McDonald's executives knew they had to at least try to figure out how to capitalize on it.

John Cisna

The first hint of a gesture came from the president of McDonald's USA, Jeff Stratton, who invited me, along with the three main students who helped me with my experiment and their parents, for an all-expenses-paid trip to McDonald's headquarters outside Chicago. We got a VIP tour of Hamburger University, fantastic hotel accommodations, and the rock-star treatment from pretty much everyone we met.

When I met Jeff Stratton for the first time in Chicago, he had a big smile on his face. He told me that McDonald's had been struggling with a certain media issue, which disappeared when I came along and did all those shows in New York.

"John, you were manna from heaven!" he said. This was the first time it really hit me how big my little experiment was for McDonald's. Later on, I found out that Jeff Stratton had been at a conference with many owner/operators after my story went viral and they all asked him what he intended to do with John Cisna. Apparently, he told them that they were working on bringing me on board, but he never tipped his hand at our first meeting.

Toward the end of that day Jeff asked if my wife and I would be willing to be his guests at the next McDonald's World Wide Convention in Orlando, Florida. I happily accepted his invitation, knowing that I'd have to juggle some things with my employer back in Iowa. I played it cool with Jeff Stratton, but I was doing cartwheels in my mind.

An Unconventional Convention

The first book I wrote, *My McDonald's Diet*, was ready for release just before I went to the McDonald's World Wide Convention. In speaking with Jeff Stratton, I mentioned that it might be cool to bring the book down with me to sell to the owner/operators.

He went one better and told me that he'd buy 1,000 copies from me directly, then set me up at a table to sign books for people who would donate twenty dollars to Ronald McDonald House Charities.

When I got to the convention it was pretty unbelievable. I saw life-size cutouts of me all around the convention center promoting my book signings.

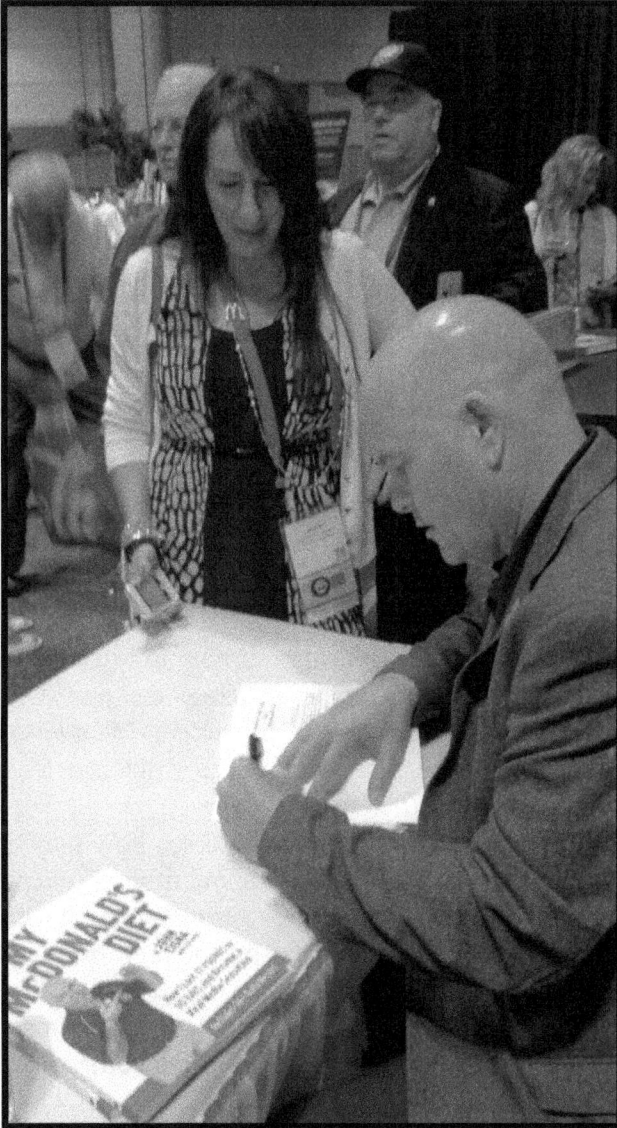

People lined up to meet me and buy my book at the
McDonald's World Wide Convention in 2014.

John Cisna

I literally had to pinch myself. One day I'm a nobody teaching school and the next day I'm a celebrity of sorts. When I got to my first book signing, I couldn't believe the interest. The line was a hundred feet long for the entire three hours, and folks were buying ten and twenty books at a time. It got so busy that people had to give me lists of who they wanted their books signed to so I could do the actual signing later and have them pick up the books the following day.

Everyone who came up to me at those signings, and elsewhere during the convention, were simply incredible and poured out their gratitude for my story and me. I have to admit, however, that it got kind of scary. I was walking around a convention center with 17,000 people who were very curious about me. They wanted autographs and pictures taken with me. It was pretty surreal!

My wife Kim and I were treated like royalty the whole time, and toward the end of the conference we got to sit next to President Stratton in the front row of an Adam Levine and Sting concert. We were totally blown away by the whole experience.

A Brand Ambassador Is Born

As I found out later, figuring out how to bring me on wasn't the easiest decision for McDonald's. While the president and the owner/operators were pushing for it, several people within the company had their doubts. I was some hick science teacher from Iowa—would I screw it up?

The company hired focus groups to see how they could best utilize me. And after I passed that test, some of the best creative and strategic minds within the company were put on the case. They knew that the microscopes would be on them from all angles and they wanted to do this right if they were going to make a commitment to me. They came to the conclusion that this should be a grassroots, local-level campaign focused on getting my message into different schools instead of some big, flashy media campaign. It really made no difference to me, but I should say that I was a lot happier talking to live audiences than I would have been shooting commercials.

On July 1, 2014, two months after my trip to McDonald's headquarters, I signed an agreement to be a brand ambassador for McDonald's. This was totally new to the fast-food chain, and it was totally new to me.

We reached an agreement on an initial one-year deal. I was an independent contractor, and I charged a fee every time I was booked to make a speech or an appearance. I wasn't on the McDonald's payroll and didn't receive any benefits like insurance or anything like that. I wasn't even eligible for an employee discount! I got a 1099 Form at the end of the year showing the amount I was paid, and I was responsible for paying my own taxes.

My status as a contractor/consultant was important for everyone, because people needed to know that I was independent of McDonald's and not acting as a puppet on a string. When I was giving speeches, they were about my experiment, my conclusions, and my story. And when I wasn't traveling for McDonald's, I was employed back home by the Des Moines Public Schools as a substitute teacher.

Class Acts: The Owner/Operators

Without a doubt, the success of my brand ambassadorship was due to the countless owner/ operators of McDonald's throughout the country who drew inspiration and energy from my story. The most enjoyable part of my relationship with McDonald's was getting to know these dedicated, hardworking people who drive, according to a BBC report published in 2012, the world's second largest private employer behind Walmart, with annual revenue around twenty-five billion dollars.

I've been to hundreds of McDonald's restaurants across this great country of ours, and I've never met a single owner/operator who wasn't among the most genuine, caring, and giving individuals I had ever met. If the fast-food critics of the world could have the kind of experiences I had with these people, they might think twice about their narrow views of the industry.

I can't speak highly enough of the incredible people who invest in McDonald's franchises. They were literally under siege by the movie *Super Size Me*, and they truly saw my existence as a way to finally show how ridiculous that darn documentary really was.

During the first six months of my brand ambassadorship, McDonald's sent me to speak in front of regional co-op meetings. These gatherings consisted of owner/operators, managers, and other executives at the local level. This is where I really got to dip my toe in the water to see how my presentation would be received.

The largest group I had ever spoken to prior to signing a contract with McDonald's was probably a classroom with thirty kids. Now all of a sudden, I found myself addressing audiences of between four hundred and eight hundred people.

My very first experience before a large audience was in Dallas, Texas. When I walked on stage and saw fourteen hundred eyes staring at me, I remember thinking, "We aren't in Kansas anymore."

I simply told my story—without a teleprompter—and tried to remain inside the general outline I had created for the presentation. I spoke factually, but also from the heart. In fact, I went out on a limb and exposed my soul to this group by saying, "This experiment has saved my life!"

When I was done, seven hundred people stood on their feet and gave me the loudest ovation I could ever imagine. I thought my presentation would be well received by a friendly crowd of McDonald's executives and employees, but I had no idea it would have this kind of an impact.

That's when it really hit me that this was something special for the owner/operators of McDonald's. In every venue over the next six months I got the same response. Standing ovation after standing ovation. I have an ego as wide as Iowa and my wife was constantly reminding me to keep this in perspective and not let it go to my head.

I tried to stay grounded, and with the help of people who really knew me, I was able to keep it fairly under control. You can't begin to imagine the adrenaline rush when you get that type of response from your fellow human beings. It's a feeling I'll never forget to my dying day.

As I continued to get an overwhelming response from audiences with direct connections to McDonald's, more people started pushing for my story to get outside the corporation and into the community. Soon after, local ad agencies started scheduling me to speak at a wide variety of civic organizations, especially schools. In 2015, I must have traveled at least 120,000 miles and spoke to well over 150,000 students ranging from ages twelve to twenty-two. And in every town I went to, I had interviews with reporters, radio hosts, and news anchors.

One of the most efficient parts of the McDonald's operation is the way the company coordinates with ad agencies in local markets. McDonald's is so big that having a single, national agency would make logistics very difficult. Having local agencies that understand the people in those areas makes tons of sense, and I witnessed first hand how well this process works.

The local agencies work directly with the local McDonald's co-op groups of owner/operators in each region. When the owner/operators make a request, like when they asked me to speak to them, the local agencies are called in to coordinate logistics. In my case, an agency would send a formal request to the corporate communications team for approval. It would include what they wanted me to do and my press availability. This was extremely efficient, as requests for my speaking in some months would require me to be gone eighteen to twenty days.

If someone asked me directly to appear, I'd simply point them to my handlers and let them take it from there. Once scheduled, it became the responsibility of the local agency to facilitate the speaking engagements, along with corresponding media appearances and interviews.

Everywhere I went a local agency rep would be there with me. I got to know these reps very well, which made being on the road a lot more fun.

The Communication Wranglers

Aside from the advice of my loving wife, I encountered a few other things that helped keep me humble, including the group of handlers who were assigned to me from the McDonald's communications team. They had their work cut out for them because they had to make sure I didn't say anything stupid.

John Cisna

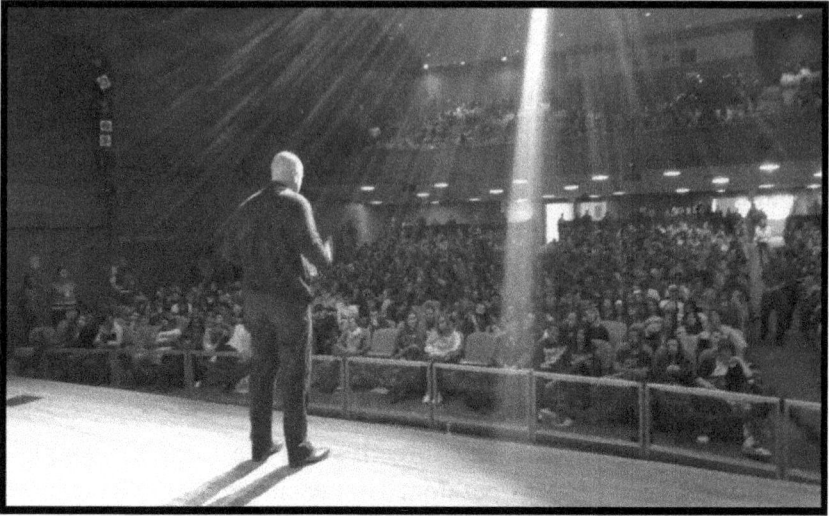

I loved getting up in front of an audience and telling my story.
I'm a natural-born motivator!

Very quickly it became clear to me that speaking on behalf of a large and highly regulated business organization was a lot different than speaking off the cuff in a television studio as the latest media curiosity. When it was just me I could say what I wanted, talk to whoever I wanted, and post whatever I wanted on social media. But when I started representing McDonald's—even though I was technically independent—it quickly became apparent that I was going to be put on a short leash.

Admittedly, this was a bit frustrating for a guy who can't help but shoot from the hip sometimes, but I understood that my handlers had to be careful that I didn't say or do something that would get them into trouble.

I'm just a regular guy and the corporate executives at McDonald's just weren't used to such an animal, but the people on the communications team worked hard to get my presentation as buttoned up as possible. I'm the kind of guy who just likes to wing it, but McDonald's wanted everything scripted and followed to the letter. Millions of people were going to be watching everything I said and did, and my corporate sponsor was ultimately responsible. McDonald's had never had to deal with anything quite like me. They had to be ever so careful in sending me out to speak publicly to make sure I didn't damage the image of McDonald's with something I might inadvertently say.

One of the biggest frustrations for me, which I know was also true for the communications team at McDonald's, was learning to change my small-town ways. I was an everyday, regular guy from a small town in Iowa who didn't have to think very much about being politically correct or worry about the impact of a unintentional statement that might offend someone else. That is the kind of scrutiny that McDonald's has to live with every day in our overly litigious society.

For the entire first year of my speaking engagements, McDonald's sent a representative from the communications team with me for every event. During my first three or four months on the road, the communications team evaluated my presentations and provided me with a list of changes. Do this. Don't say that.

These weren't big changes to the story. They were little nitpicky changes to some examples I used that my millennial handlers considered definite no-no's. My response to their recommendations was usually a very sincere, "Are you kidding me?!"

One thing they asked me to take out was my ice-breaking magic trick. I've been an amateur magician for forty years, and crowds are always entertained by the tricks I do. They get a good laugh and loosen up. But the communications team thought that audiences would think my whole experiment was an illusion if I started off with a little sleight of hand. ARE YOU KIDDING ME?!

Another thing they took out of my presentation was a story I told to illustrate how impressionable young people are, and how they'll tend to believe anything, without looking into the facts, if it comes from someone with authority. Early in my teaching career, I nearly had two seventh graders convinced that white cows produced regular milk and black cows produced chocolate milk. The communications team decided that this could be taken as a racist comment. ARE YOU KIDDING ME?!

Someone asked me in a question and answer session how I deal with people who simply refuse to believe the results of my experiment. My reply was, "Look, some people have made up their minds that cannot be changed no matter what proof is shown. There are still people today who believe the Holocaust never happened." I was told never to say that again because it would be offensive to Jewish people. ARE YOU KIDDING ME?!

To the McDonald's folks, I was a wild card with little to no filter between my brain and my lips. I spoke my mind, political correctness be damned. The team from McDonald's was just trying to mitigate any potential disaster from an offhand comment.

To their credit, they never told me how to tell my story. With the exception of a few word tweaks here and there, they never intervened with the core of my presentation.

McDonald's had every incentive for our relationship to work. And, I have to say, in my first year as a McDonald's brand ambassador, the company treated me embarrassingly well. Here I was a simple science teacher from a small town with a simple experiment that sent shockwaves around the globe with mind-blowing empirical data. Company executives were thrilled that they finally had something concrete to counter *Super Size Me,* and, more importantly, get into the classroom to educate students that what you ate was more important than where you ate.

McDonald's treated me like a rock star. They had cars waiting to whisk me away to and from every appearance. They put me up in some of the nicest hotels I've ever stayed at. They paid for my food. They did everything they could to make sure I focused on engaging and entertaining the crowds that came to see me.

The Video That Almost Undid Me

Over the years, corporate McDonald's had been trying to persuade the local owner/operators to get into the schools, and now they had a golden opportunity.

As I mentioned earlier, a wrench was thrown into my brand ambassadorship when a woman who blogs about food and kids came after me. What really got her goat, however, was a video that McDonald's made to chronicle my experiment. The twenty-nine minute documentary was a professionally produced film called *540 Meals*, which was the number of McDonald's meals I ate over the course of six months.

The video was available for viewing online, and it was pitched to schools as part of my educational program. Schools that invited me to speak also got the video, along with an educational discussion guide. The film would be screened, and then I'd come out and talk for another thirty minutes or so.

The film was fine, but I was a little upset that McDonald's just went ahead and made it without my involvement. I fancy myself a bit of a video editor and I put together my own documentary of my original experiment.

Once the news of my project went viral, many teachers across the country asked if I had anything I could share with them about the project. Of course, I had my video, and I sent the link to dozens of colleagues who used it in their classrooms.

My original intention was to get *Super Size Me* out of the classroom and my documentary into the classroom, or at least convince other educators to show both films and generate a lively discussion that allowed kids to use and develop valuable critical thinking skills.

My video, like me, is down-to-earth, data driven, and funny at times. And I filled it up with a lot of student interviews so more kids could relate to it.

You can view my video *The "McDonalds" Project* today if you want to at https://youtu.be/VdDISVIbn1o. I hope you enjoy it.

McDonald's, however, didn't much like my video. They thought it wasn't professional enough, but that was its charm and the corporate suits completely missed it. They told me that my video violated all kinds of FTC rules and regulations, and assured me that the video they were going to make on their own would be a thousand times better.

They suggested that they might use some of my footage (they didn't), but I had absolutely no say in how the new video would be created or used. That was that.

A few weeks later, a husband-and-wife film crew came to Iowa to interview a few other teachers and me, and to get B-roll of my school. It was kind of funny when I met them. They flew into Des Moines from New York and I picked them up at the airport to drive them to Colo, about forty-five minutes northeast. For the longest time, they just stared out the window and didn't say a word.

John Cisna

It was fall, you see, and they just couldn't believe how the abundant cornfields stretched out into infinity in every direction. They definitely weren't in New York City anymore!

The filmmakers were selected by winning a creative pitch through a company called Tongal. The film they ended up making, the soon-to-be-infamous *540 Meals*, was recognized by the Tongal family of affiliated filmmakers with a prestigious "Tongie" award.

About three weeks after the filmmakers left Iowa, I received a link to watch *540 Meals* in all its nineteen minutes of glory. While the production was slick and the interviews came off good, I couldn't believe that they took out a critical element of my entire experiment—my before and after blood work. This was the thing that really showed the improved "healthiness" that had occurred from eating all that fast food.

I was pretty vocal about how upset this made me, and I told my handlers on the communication team, and anyone else who'd listen, that if they sent me out into the world without the ability to show my blood work results, the press would eat me alive.

After much whining, and with support from various owner/operators, McDonald's finally relented and put my blood results into the video.

I'm glad they finally listened to me, but in the scheme of things it didn't really mean much. The whole video and discussion guide were out of my hands. Even though I had more than eight years of experience as a high school teacher, I was never asked to contribute to those pieces! It was what it was, and that's what we were going with, so I didn't put up a stink about it anymore after the blood work was edited in.

I had a lot of other things on my mind anyway, like the half-hour presentation I had to give. Fortunately, our first stop was in Tampa, Florida, to spend some time with an owner/operator named Blake Casper. Blake tracked me down right after my story went viral, and when I was still a full-time teacher, I spoke to his group and got a big standing ovation. Blake is a big deal in the McDonald's organization. He owns fifty-four restaurants and has his own distribution center to make sure his locations have all the ingredients and supplies they need to run efficiently and profitably.

I tried my new speech on his group and it was met with thunderous applause. The video was pretty well received, too, so I didn't think much more about it. And everywhere we went, whether we were speaking to schools or to owner/operator meetings, the applause was deafening and the chairs must have all had springs in them. In Dallas, six hundred people stood up for me. In Phoenix, another five hundred people. Same thing in Denver. It was really nice, but also a little scary. I can see how that kind of adulation can get to you, and maybe what was about to happen with the food advocate was designed to keep me humble!

My "Advocate" in Houston

In the fall of 2015, I think it was October, the communications team called to warn me about something. There was a woman in Houston, Texas, named Bettina Siegel who headed a blog group called lunchtray.com. My handlers informed me that they had run across this lady in years past, and that she basically hated McDonald's and everything it stood for.

She and her tens of thousands of followers were hell-bent on blasting McDonald's and me for trying to convince people to eat more fast food, especially McDonald's.

What she was really objecting to was *540 Meals* and the associated educational packet that went along with it, since she had never seen my presentation nor discussed any of these issues with me directly.

Honestly, I would have loved to have talked with her or any of my critics. I would have told them what kind of response we got at every school we visited. I would have shown her the testimonials we videotaped showing that the main message people got out of *540 Meals* and my talk was one of accountability and choice. Not once did anyone tell me they were going to start eating more fast food!

What disappointed me the most about my critics were the assumptions they seemed to be making about students. My critics never seemed to give the young people who heard my message any credit as critical thinkers, which was the whole point of my experiment. Rather than shut my program down, I believe that my critics would have been better served to work with McDonald's and

31

me to make sure the message of choice and accountability for one's actions came through loud and clear.

I was offering a simple message about the importance of choice—with food and other aspects of life—and nothing else. Anyone who had seen my presentation understood that. If any of the critics had simply taken the time to watch the presentation or talk with me directly, this controversy would have been greatly minimized.

Bettina Siegel is a self-described food advocate who shut me down and still proudly touts her attack on my presentation with McDonald's. Her attack against me began when she featured a story on her website about "540 Meals: Choices Make the Difference." She believed the video was being presented as a "nutrition education" program, when it was nothing more than a nineteen-minute McDonald's commercial.

Thanks to a large following and an assist by the *Washington Post*, Siegel convinced ninety thousand people to sign her petition to stop me from visiting middle and high schools across the country.

She appealed to the parents' natural concern for their children's welfare, calling the film a "naked advertising effort" designed to manipulate "impressionable kids."

This paragraph from her change.org petition pretty much sums it all up:

> ***Teens and pre-teens are notoriously impulsive***. *So when a trusted authority like a science teacher says he ate fries on a near-daily basis for six months, as well as regularly eating Big Macs, Quarter Pounders and ice cream—and that he still eats at McDonald's every day—do we think teens are suddenly going to become highly disciplined calorie-cutters? Or do we think they'll get the message that it's OK to eat even more fast food?*

I just wish she had gotten her facts straight and maybe even talked to me. But she didn't. And, in the interest of full disclosure, McDonald's wouldn't have let me near her even if she did reach out to me.

Instead, she made me out to be a liar by taking things out of context. In an October 12, 2015, article about me, she confuses a statement I made about having my students plan all my meals by saying they came up with the idea for the experiment. In the same piece, she goes on to say that I never specified the fifteen nutrients I tracked in my research when I clearly do on page 15 of my first book, and which McDonald's clearly did in *540 Meals*. I also mentioned them every time I gave a presentation, and even pointed out that the students who planned my meals couldn't come close to staying inside the FDA guidelines of sodium. I did not, as she claimed, "deliberately [omit] sodium from the mix, even though it's one of the main 'nutrients of concern' in the American diet." She accused me of "nutrient cherry-picking," but that was nothing but fake news.

One thing Ms. Siegel wrote was true, and that's the fact that no one from McDonald's agreed to talk to her about my presentation or me. I wish they had, and I wish they had let me respond to her directly—and to the countless hateful tweets and emails I got from her followers. I still get messages today from people saying things like they hope I die. And now that I have the freedom to respond, I politely explain what really went down, and I either get a thank-you note or never hear from them again.

When you really boil the whole thing down, I believe that Ms. Siegel's biggest concern—outside of the fact that McDonald's was allowed onto school property at all—was that the *540 Meals* video was positioned as an educational program and contained language that said, "There's nothing wrong with fast food. There's nothing wrong with McDonald's."

Ms. Siegel wrote that "even in the midst of a childhood obesity epidemic, *540 Meals* irresponsibly encourages notoriously impulsive pre-teen and teenaged kids to frequent McDonald's—with all of its powerful sensory cues and unhealthful offerings—even more often than they already do."

She railed at the film for being propaganda, and complained that it should have contained language that stated something like "your calorie needs may be significantly lower than John Cisna's," as well as information about calculating one's daily caloric requirements.

Look, I have my own problems with the materials McDonald's created to accompany my presentations, but I think Ms.

Siegel is unfair in her assessment of them. Right in the middle of *540 Meals*, I'm on camera saying, "I would never recommend that anyone eat only McDonald's all day, every day for months. But my story demonstrates that through planning and mindful choices, you can still enjoy your favorite McDonald's items and meet your goals at the same time."

And right at the end of the video, this message appears on the screen for about ten seconds, making it really hard to miss:

> *No one is suggesting that anyone should eat every meal at McDonald's or that eating at McDonald's will result in any health benefit. Rather, as John says, it's not about where you eat but the choices you make and how much you exercise.*

If you're interested, I encourage you to watch *540 Meals* and make your own decisions about how educational it is. It's not available in too many places, but as I write this it's up on YouTube at https://www.youtube.com/watch?v=jLxlU-uAHIY.

Ms. Siegel kept up her campaign against McDonald's with appearances on the *TODAY* show and *The Doctors*. In both appearances, she debated a nutritional consultant hired by McDonald's, a woman named Shaye Arluk. On *The Doctors*, Ms. Arluk said that it was important to have conversations with teenagers—40 percent of whom eat fast food on a daily basis—about how to make better choices so they can balance their nutrients and avoid eating too many calories.

While the hosts of the show said they didn't disagree with the message, their big problem was with the McDonald's branding in the *540 Meals* video. Jim Searn, MD, a pediatrician, commented that the video "is essentially a nineteen-minute infomercial for McDonald's. Thirty-six times the word McDonald's is mentioned—that's every thirty-one seconds—so that is...a heavily branded message that I don't think belongs in schools. I think the message is okay, but the fact that it's coming from McDonald's, being paid for by McDonald's, is just not the way to go."

He also said that I seem "like a cool guy." Let me tell you, I would have loved to have been a part of that show. Speaking on my behalf, however, was another cool guy named Adam Kurth, the principal of Luxemburg-CASCO High School outside Green Bay, Wisconsin. The school has a McDonald's just a hundred yards from campus, and it was one of the last schools I spoke at before the whole controversy arose.

Mr. Kurth called into the program and said that having McDonald's and me talk to his students was both positive and appropriate. On the air, he complimented me for doing a nice job of highlighting the power of our choices—not just at McDonald's but anywhere people go—and said that he expected his teachers to talk about the presentation with their students.

After he finished explaining what really happened, Ms. Siegel looked pretty foolish in my opinion. But that didn't stop her from mentioning her petition to get *540 Meals* and me out of the schools. She pointed out that Ms. Arluk admitted on camera that the video was never meant to be educational, and that while the video is fine on YouTube or in theaters, it shouldn't be in our schools.

I didn't spend a whole lot of time even worrying about this because I knew the message I was delivering in my speeches was a positive one. And, like I say in *540 Meals*, "when I hear the skeptics, it doesn't disgruntle me. It actually fires me up because those are the people that I have to educate."

In my view, Ms. Siegel and I will probably never see eye-to-eye on the fast-food issue. She's definitely entitled to her opinions, but I wish she hadn't worked so hard to stop a program that I believe was having a positive impact on students across the country.

In my presentation, I always told students to take whatever they hear or read, especially on the Internet, with a healthy dose of skepticism. I encouraged them to always investigate all the facts and make as informed a decision as possible.

But all that was overlooked in Ms. Siegel's effort to get McDonald's out of school auditoriums and classrooms. The things she told her followers about me led to some very personal attacks on social media:

"You call yourself a teacher?"

"You ought to be ashamed of yourself."

John Cisna

"You are a piece of s***."

And the tweet I'll never forget: "What John Cisna is doing to young people's' minds is worse than what Jared did but on a bigger scale."

These tweets were so vicious that being mad never really crossed my mind. What I really thought about was how sad these people's lives were that they would say such things about me without ever meeting me, seeing me, hearing me, or even writing to me to investigate the facts about what I was doing.

The few people who actually took time out of their day to throw hate at me were far outnumbered by the tens of thousands of people I spoke to during this campaign who only had positive reactions to my message of personal responsibility and me. Bill Murray, the comedian, conveyed it best when he said, "Winning an argument against an intelligent person is very difficult. Winning an argument against a stupid person is damn near impossible."

The Doctors show, which took place in December 2015, ended up being the nail in the coffin that put an end to my message being delivered in schools across the country. I gave my last speech in a school in March 2016 and received yet another wonderful response from students, teachers, and administrators.

In my view, it's really a shame that Ms. Siegel and I never connected. Who knows, maybe we could have joined forces in some way. I know it sounds kind of crazy, but in a way we're both trying to do the same thing by educating kids on how to make better choices about their health.

I just needed a hook to get people interested in what I was doing, and that hook was McDonald's. If I had just told my students to put me on a 2,000-calorie-per-day diet and keep my nutrients close to the FDA recommended daily allowances, I wouldn't have created much news—even in the school paper! And tens of thousands of kids across the country would never have received my positive message of choice and accountability.

I often referred to McDonald's at that time as my grocery store. And that particular grocery store put severe limits on the students who were tasked to create my daily menus. That was the whole point of the experiment—to help kids use their critical thinking skills and apply deductive reasoning to make the best choices possible with the resources they had to deal with.

Isn't this what we all want for our children? Shame on me for trying to get these kids to think for themselves. Shame on me for not simply dictating what they should eat. Shame on me for introducing the results of an experiment that should make all of us take a second look at how we view food. Shame on me for even suggesting that we should be responsible for our own choices.

If sophomores in high school can make their fat, overweight, out-of-shape, heart-attack-waiting-to-happen teacher healthier than when he started eating nothing but fast food, think of what they could do with a wider selection of food like we have in this country. I really believe that my students, and the majority of the students that I had the honor of speaking to as a McDonald's brand ambassador, are making healthier choices today because of my McDonald's experiment.

I was definitely upset when I could no longer speak to students, largely because the uproar was mostly based on the *540 Meals* video taken out of context. The part of the program where I go on stage and talk directly to the audience was a lot more nuanced than the film, but my presentation was glossed over and treated by people with no knowledge of it as more of the same. I went to great lengths in my presentation to say that while weight loss is a function of calories in versus calories out, the kind of calories that go in are really important.

Please hear me loudly when I say that WEIGHT LOSS BY ITSELF IS NOT AN INDICATOR OF GETTING HEALTHY. If, instead of eating at McDonald's, I consumed eight Milky Way bars a day (about 2,000 calories), I still would have lost weight, but I might have died of sugar shock before the three months were up.

Validation from Another Group of Doctors

After *The Doctors* show and McDonald's decision to pull me out of the schools, my schedule got a lot less hectic. I was still speaking at Rotary Club functions, insurance luncheons, and other community events, and I even got the opportunity to be the keynote

John Cisna

speaker at the 100th anniversary of the Utah Public Health Convention.

I was a little snake bit after the whole Bettina Siegel campaign, and I was a little nervous about this particular presentation. How appropriate, I thought, that one of my last appearances for McDonald's would be in front of several hundred physicians, dietitians, nutritionists, and PhDs who all forgot more about health than I ever learned in my lifetime.

If my story and presentation were truly not right, this group would overwhelmingly let me have it. I didn't change a thing in my presentation and I got a very warm round of applause at the end. I felt pretty good that no one booed me off the stage, heckled me, or threw rotten tomatoes at me.

One lady came up to me afterward and told me she was going to use my story as part of her PhD dissertation on food and obesity.

About a month later, I received the results of a survey that the Utah Public Health Department had given to the people who attended my presentation. I knew what was in the envelope and took a deep breath before opening it, and I almost started to cry when I saw the results.

These educated health professionals had overwhelmingly responded to my presentation just as I hoped they would. They understood the value of personal accountability and why it's so important for us to teach children how to look at the facts and make their own best, informed decisions.

On all eight questions, the number of "Agree" and "Strongly Agree" responses were overwhelming:

Question	Agree/Strongly Agree Response Percentage
The presenter addressed the learning objective.	92.10%
The presenter demonstrated mastery of the subject.	84.21%
The presenter was responsive to participants.	89.48%

The presenter's teaching methods and style held my attention.	92.10%
The presentation content had substance.	76.31%
The presentation was current and relevant.	81.58%
I would like to learn more about this topic.	63.16%
I would like to hear this presenter again.	63.16%

2016 Utah Conference for Public Health
Presenter Evaluation, John Cisna

Many of the specific comments I received from conference attendees were also gratifying:

"Bold move that paid off."

"I thought this was a very interesting presentation—I like that it kind of "ruffled" a few feathers and made people think a bit harder."

"The presenter was phenomenal. I didn't realize he's been speaking for an hour when his time was up."

"I loved this presentation.... This is how we should all discuss topics on which we may not totally see eye-to-eye. Great job on having the guts to invite Mr. Cisna to this event."

"Outstanding, I'm so pleased UPHA is bringing in thought-provoking speakers. I get tired of the organization bringing in safe (and boring) speakers. It is thinking outside the box. LOVE it and makes me want to continue being a member."

"I think his presentation was great. I have seen him speak before and it was really similar. His message is about making choices and shows the science behind weight loss—it is a balance of calories burned vs. consumed. I

know some people didn't appreciate this talk. However, I think the dialogue it has created is important. We need to be able to discuss ideas that are different from our own. Of course, I would never advocate a McDonald's diet, he isn't advocating that either. But I think there are a lot of takeaways from his message, such as the power of choice and mindful eating that are extremely valuable to our field. Most Americans don't care about what data some highly educated health scientists present. They can, however, relate to a middle school science teacher who found a way to lose weight while teaching his students in the process."

After battling Bettina Siegel for months, it was nice to get some positive feedback from a room full of doctors who understood the real point of my experiment and didn't have an axe to grind against McDonald's.

A Tattoo to Renew

Before, during, and even after the whole school hullabaloo, I worked very hard to prove my worth to McDonald's. I had given up my career in teaching to be at the fast-food chain's beck and call, which was especially risky because I didn't think I'd be able to get another teaching job if the McDonald's gig didn't work out. At fifty-five, I was at an age when most of my colleagues were retiring, or at least thinking about it.

My first brand ambassador contract was for twelve months and I was hopeful that it would be renewed for at least another year. My wish came true in the spring of 2015 when McDonald's extended our relationship for another eighteen months through calendar year 2016. The momentum of the campaign internally and in the media was huge, and McDonald's was reaping the benefits of my enthusiasm, wit, and empirical data. My story wouldn't die, and everywhere I went I created a "wow" factor that really inspired and energized my audiences.

In my wildest dreams I never thought that my simple experiment would have become a worldwide, viral sensation. I can honestly say that the whole experience has been one of the most blessed things that has ever happened to me on my life's journey. Not only was the arrangement very good financially, but it also allowed me to accomplish some of the goals I had when I decided to leave the business world in 2010 and go back into teaching.

Deep down, I've always wanted to make a difference in people's lives. I was able to do that as a teacher, which was much more fulfilling than being in sales and management, but my McDonald's experiment took it to a much higher level. I was able to speak directly to hundreds of thousands of people, and reach millions more through media reports and interviews.

When my brand ambassador contract was first coming up for renewal, I told my wife Kim that if they kept me on, I wanted to do something that would remind me forever of how fortunate I had been. About three months prior to the end of the initial agreement, I decided I was going to get some ink on my arm if they inked another deal with me—I was going to get a McDonald's tattoo.

Before I put a big yellow McDonald's "M" on my upper left arm, I never really understood why people got tattoos. Did it not cross their minds that whatever they decided (usually at a younger age) to put on their bodies would remain with them for the rest of their lives? I now understand that's exactly what people who get tattoos are most aware of. Tattoos tell stories, and most everyone represents something of importance in someone's life. My tattoo is the same: It's a constant reminder of what this little experiment brought to my life and of the responsibility I have as a human being to make a difference every day.

When I was sitting in the tattoo parlor, a woman came up to me about halfway through the process. "Is that a McDonald's tattoo?" she asked with great curiosity.

"Yes, that's correct," I said.

"Can I ask you a personal question?"

"Sure," I replied.

"Did you lose a bet?"

I thought I was going to fall off my chair laughing, and it got me to thinking that I'd love to be a mouse in the corner of the funeral home when I'm being laid to rest and the director has me on the table and says, "Hey, Charlie, come get a look at this!"

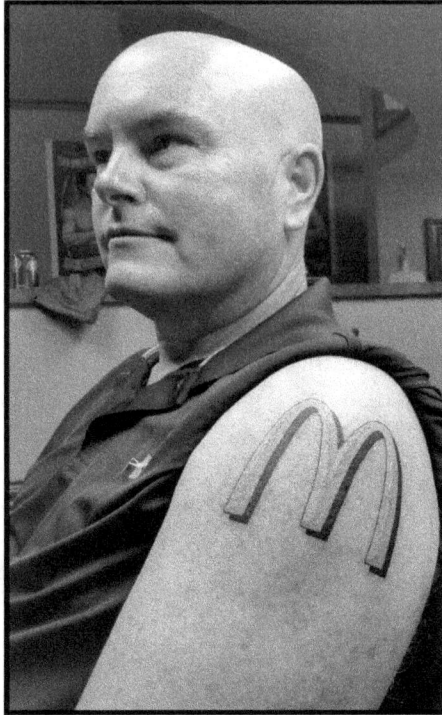

I got a McDonald's tattoo when my contract
was renewed for another year and a half.

A Breath of Fresh Air

At the end of my first year as a brand ambassador, McDonald's did some reorganizing, and I was assigned to a new person on the communications team. I didn't think this was going to affect me much since by then all the seemingly offensive parts of my presentation had been eliminated and I was being a pretty good boy. The show was basically on autopilot after twelve months of practicing and tweaking.

My new handler was a woman named Julie Barberio, who had previously worked for an owner/operator in North Carolina. Although she was new to the McDonald's corporate office, she understood the organization very well and turned out to be the best thing that could've happened to me.

Julie is a little bundle of positive energy that radiates like an atomic bomb. Have you ever seen someone enter a room and immediately say to yourself, "I want to be around that person?" That's the kind of person she is, and we really hit it off right from the start.

On our first road trip together, I knew that Julie was going to help me take my presentation to a new level. She studied crowd reactions every time I made an appearance, and she'd sit down with me afterward and share her observations while they were still fresh in her mind. We started adding a little bit here, taking a little bit from there, bringing certain points home in more compelling ways, and making the presentation better and better every time.

She also suggested that we interview teachers, principals, and superintendents at the schools after each presentation to get their impressions of what they had heard. We created a vast video library of testimonials from educators across the country, all talking about what a great message I was teaching kids about choice and accountability.

On one of our trips to Florida, she interviewed me and asked specific questions that helped drive home the point even more about how my presentation was all about developing critical thinking and deductive reasoning skills, not about building an entire diet around fast food.

Even though the communications team and McDonald's marketing people decided not to use these videos, they really helped focus my message and helped me do a better job as a brand ambassador. It was a little frustrating, but neither Julie nor I had any say in how McDonald's ran their marketing program. We just did the best jobs we could with the things we could control ourselves.

The End of an Era

Julie and I were together for the whole school controversy, and when that ended in the spring of 2016, I had the sense that it was the beginning of the end for my relationship with McDonald's and me.

My speaking schedule was limited to McDonald's groups and community organizations, and instead of traveling three or four days a week, I was down to about one or two days a month. The media appearances and interviews were drying up as well, and I knew that the powers that be at McDonald's were just trying to wind my brand ambassadorship down with as little public exposure as possible.

In the final weeks, we were all just waiting for the contract to officially end on December 31, 2016. My final call with my team occurred a few days before the end of the year. They thanked me for everything and I thanked them, and in about five minutes that was that. What started out with a bang, ended with a whimper.

I was philosophical about it. All good things come to an end, and this was definitely a good thing. I have nothing but appreciation for McDonald's for giving me the opportunity of a lifetime. I believed we reached a lot of people in a positive way, and I grew tremendously as a person in those two and a half years.

I learned a great deal about the true nature of people, and about the importance of patience when dealing with ignorance. I gained insights into the problem of food addiction, and how much of a real issue it is among thousands of people who desperately want to live healthier, but can't.

All of this has given me the fire to try to do what I can to help people in their search for a better life. I want others to experience how great life really can be when you make healthier choices. I had gained so much knowledge and enthusiasm as a McDonald's brand ambassador that I had to figure out a new way to help people be their best.

Chapter Three

A New Experiment: Fit at Fifty-Eight

My presentation at the Utah Public Health Convention was pretty much my last hurrah with McDonald's. I definitely had mixed emotions about that event because it went so well and yet I knew my time in the spotlight with McDonald's was winding down. I felt like we really had one of the greatest health and wellness messages out there, and now fewer people were going to be exposed to it.

I suppose I'm somewhat biased when I say how powerful my message of choice and responsibility is, but the responses I've gotten from people—especially those who've dealt with weight issues as I have—have confirmed that the lessons learned from my McDonald's experiment really can make a difference in people's lives. If McDonald's was no longer going to provide me with a platform to get my message out, I had to figure out how I could take it to the next level on my own.

During the last couple months of 2016, pretty much around the holidays, I took a total break from everything and put some weight back on. I didn't want to get up to the 280 pounds I was four years ago, but it felt good to let myself go for a while. It gave me a chance to separate from the headiness of my McDonald's adventure and think about what to do next. It was almost as if I had to go back to being my real self for a while before I could decide what my future was going to look like.

I definitely wanted to keep my options open. Going back into teaching wasn't practical, but I didn't have enough money to retire on. And because my wife Kim was thriving in a career she loved, and our kids were still in college, we weren't ready to live our dream of moving to Scottsdale, Arizona, quite yet. So I had to think of something to do to keep busy in Iowa, at least for the foreseeable future.

Since I know my town so well, and since I enjoy talking to people, I decided to get a broker's license and try my hand at selling real estate. I enjoyed having something to focus on, but I continued to gain weight as the McDonald's chapter of my life became more of a distant memory. I was making bad food choices again, and before I knew it I had chunked up to about 255 pounds.

Muscle Bound for Glory

Even though the idea of getting into really good shape was always in the back of my mind, I wasn't moving mountains to get on a new diet and exercise program. Quite the opposite—I was moving mountains of food into my mouth again!

One fateful Monday in January 2017, I decided to go to the weekly sales meeting at my real estate office. These meetings are optional, but since I was the new guy on the block, I tried to go as often as possible. On this particular day, I really didn't want to get my butt out of bed and go into the office, but at the last minute I decided that I NEEDED to be there.

Occasionally, in addition to the regular sales meetings, the management at my brokerage brings in guest speakers to discuss general self-help topics, ranging from improving performance to just being a better person. These informal meetings were usually fun and informative, and they were usually kept short, so people could get on with their day and get to work.

On that particular Monday, the guy who came to talk to us was someone named Brian Gaumer. He used to sell real estate for the company, but that wasn't why he came to see us. He was there to promote his new gym, a place called MuscleBoundUSA.

Just by looking at Brian, I could tell that he was in pretty good shape for a guy about my age. He was bald like me, and if we were the same height, I could have been his "before" picture! It turns out that Brian used to be a competitive bodybuilder in the 1970s when Arnold Schwarzenegger and *Pumping Iron* were bringing bodybuilding into the mainstream. He was actually Mr. Teen Iowa back in the 1970s, and came pretty close to qualifying for various Mr. USA competitions during his prime.

When I met him, he still had broad shoulders, huge arms, and washboard abs, even though he claims that he hasn't done a single sit-up or crunch in decades. And he's still incredibly strong. At the ripe old age of fifty-eight, he can deadlift more than 500 pounds. The motto for his gym, and his entire philosophy of life, is "Age don't matter!" and he seriously practices what he preaches.

During the little gathering at the real estate office, Brian spoke passionately about how a simple exercise program, along with a plant-based food plan, can do incredible things for people, especially those like me who've put their bodies through the wringer.

I really did feel like he was speaking directly to me, and because this literally fell into my lap, I decided to check out his gym after work and see what it was all about.

When I got to his place of business, I have to admit I was a little turned off by the MuscleBoundUSA sign that screamed out at the parking lot and the street beyond. I was afraid I was going to walk into the place and find a bunch of lunkheads posing and flexing in Speedos. That was definitely not what I was looking for, but I still went in with as open a mind as I could muster.

Brian recognized me from the meeting that morning. After we talked for a bit, he immediately remembered my McDonald's project and all its associated frenzy. I told him I put the weight back on and was looking for a new program to get healthy again. I asked him to go into detail about this program he'd come up with.

He really caught my attention when he said, "What would happen if you could take one of the best exercise programs around and combine it with one of the best food plans?"

The answer was fairly obvious, but identifying effective exercise and dietary components that work perfectly together is a big challenge for most people. I continued to listen with great interest and became more and more excited about giving his program a try. What really sealed the deal for me was a documentary Brian told me to watch on Netflix called *Forks Over Knives*. It scared the sheep dip out of me and I signed up for Brian's program the very next day!

A month later I shared my blood work with my real estate colleagues. They were so impressed with the results that six of them signed up for Brian's program, and four of them are still doing it today. Three of them are women, so while this book talks a lot about increasing testosterone for greater health, this program isn't just for the guys.

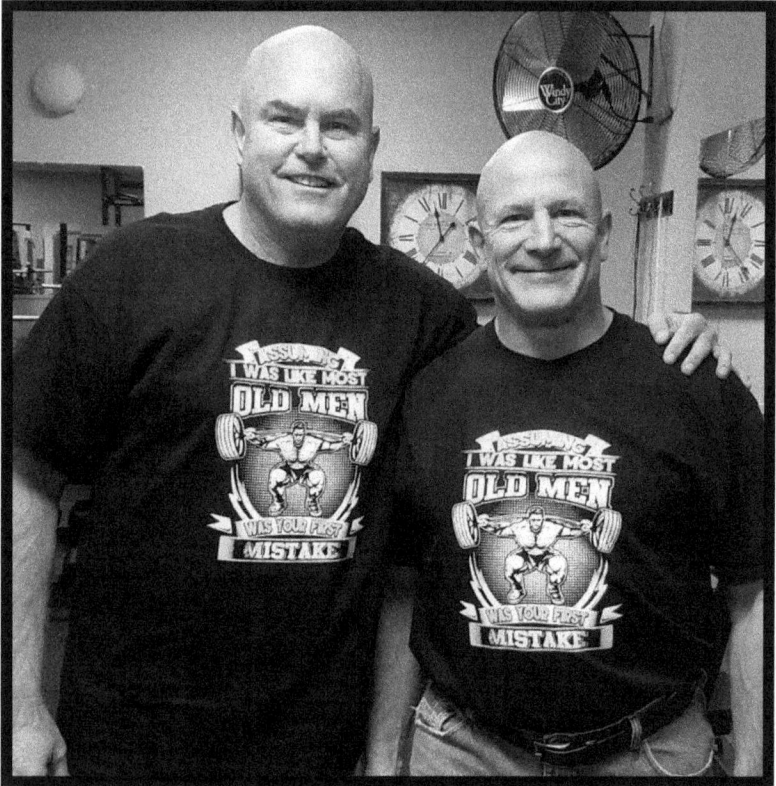

My guru, Brian Gaumer, and me at MuscleBoundUSA

Back in the Saddle

I have to confess that it felt really great to have an experiment to work on again. I guess you just can't take the scientist out of me! I really do thrive when I have a hypothesis to test. And because I really wasn't happy about being fat again, it was great that my new experiment involved changing my eating and exercise habits for the better.

As you'll read in the following pages, I followed Brian's program to a T, measured all my progress, and faithfully got my blood work done every six weeks like I did with my McDonald's experiment. And once again the data didn't lie.

I was so impressed with what this new program has done for me that I decided to write this second book about how an even BETTER set of choices has made me stronger, happier, and healthier than I've ever been before.

Back when I was fifty-three years old and weighing in at 280 pounds, I would have believed a prediction that by age fifty-eight I'd have a heart attack over another prediction that I'd be in the best shape of my life. Now I look and feel like I'm in my thirties, and I know I'm on the path to get even healthier as time goes on.

You may be thinking, "This is one guy's pipe dream that I'm not going to be able to achieve."

I'll show you how you can achieve greater health and vitality, and at a minimal cost of both dollars AND time. It sounds too good to be true, which is exactly what I thought when I was introduced to it, but I gave it a shot.

Was I worried about it failing? I NEVER worry about trying things that may fail. Success is the result of things we learn from failure. Show me a person who has never failed, and I'll show you a person who has never grown.

I've failed in many things in my lifetime, but the successes I've had are a direct result of all those misses. I'm here to tell you that, as the subtitle of this book says, the Fountain of Youth IS real, and I hope you'll take the risk of finding it for yourself.

On the following pages I'll outline the details of the incredible program I'm on, so you can decide if it's for you or not. And please know that I'm not trying to sell you anything beyond this book, which, presumably, you've already bought. I'm just here to be a human lab rat to show anyone, especially middle-aged guys, that fantastic health is possible at any age.

Chapter Four

5X5: Exercises for Strength, Muscle, and Higher T

I know now that weight training is the absolute best way to lose fat and gain strength, but I never picked up a dumbbell or a barbell until my first session at MuscleBoundUSA. Back when I played Division I baseball in the 1970s, my coaches told me not to lift weights because it would limit the flexibility I needed to throw, run, and swing. In other words, they didn't want me to get muscle bound!

Even after I got injured and stopped playing college ball, I never really even thought about exercising for health, let alone starting to lift weights. I just lifted a lot of food up to my mouth and got fat!

But Brian Gaumer was persuasive about his program, so I thought I'd give it a try. What did I have to lose? If it didn't work, I wouldn't be any worse off, and it certainly wouldn't have taken up much of my time—the strength-training program he promotes requires just forty-five minutes, three days a week.

Brian calls it the best, most efficient exercise program around, but it's more popularly known as the 5X5. The training protocol was first developed by the legendary Bill Starr, a reclusive, stubborn, and controversial figure who devoted his career to making football players, other athletes, and even regular people as strong as they could be given their individual genetics.

Starr worked for the York Barbell company as a young man, and wrote articles about weightlifting and conditioning for a magazine called *Strength and Health*. He's best known for revolutionizing the role of strength and conditioning coaches on college and professional sports teams. He worked for the Baltimore Colts when they won Super Bowl V, and he also coached athletes at the University of Hawaii, Southern Methodist University, and Johns Hopkins throughout his illustrious career.

John Cisna

The book that outlines his radical training methods is called *The Strongest Shall Survive*. Published in 1976, this 205-page manual for athletes describes Bill Starr's unique prescriptions for training, nutrition, and rehabilitation.

His basic concept was that overall strength is the primary training goal. Aesthetics can come later, but strength is the foundation.

To get stronger, all you really need are a few compound movements that work a variety of muscle groups at the same time. There's no need for a wide variety of exercises for specific body parts, also known as isolation exercises.

That's really the beauty of the program. You can cut out all those silly little exercises for your quadriceps, hamstrings, calves, chest, back, shoulders, biceps, triceps, and abs, and simply focus on a total of five core movements in specific combinations.

Mehdi or Not, Here We Come

While the 5X5 program had its devotees over the years, it never really took root in the public consciousness as the best way to get in shape. Instead, people think they have to mix things up and do tons of isolation exercises to train different muscle groups from different angles. That certainly keeps the fitness magazines chock-full of content, and it may be fine for advanced trainers looking to sculpt their physiques to look a certain way, but it's certainly not what most of us need to build a foundation of strength, health, and conditioning.

In 2007, the 5X5 method experienced a revival of sorts, thanks to a guy named Mehdi Hadim, who simply goes by his first name. Mehdi's website, stronglifts.com, gets a million hits a day, and the man is on a mission to bring this incredible exercise regimen to the masses. I've corresponded with Mehdi on several occasions and he definitely practices what he preaches.

Mehdi has attained incredible strength using the 5X5 weight-training program. He got inspired to change his life when he couldn't beat any of his friends at arm wrestling—even the girls! At the time, he couldn't even do one push up. He looked at himself in the mirror and decided that he no longer wanted to be a "skinny-fat weakling."

Mehdi gave up TV and video games for a gym membership, and started a typical weight-training routine that included different exercises for different body parts. He worked chest, back, shoulders, legs, and arms, all on different days and pushing himself to failure on every set. He was perpetually sore, wasn't getting great results, and ultimately gave it up.

He admits that he was pretty naïve at the time, not realizing that most of the people who make rapid gains on overly punishing routines are often on steroids. He definitely didn't want to go that route, but he still wanted to get strong.

Eventually, he went back to the gym and found someone who agreed to mentor him. Mehdi recalls throwing up during his first workout while doing squats, but he hung in there for two whole years and got the strength he was seeking.

But gaining that strength took Mehdi a lot of time and effort, and he also had a life to live. So about four years after he became fanatical about lifting weights, he discovered that he could get great results in less time with Bill Starr's 5X5 routine. An article he read online described the routine that legendary bodybuilder Reg Park taught to Arnold Schwarzenegger before he became larger than life—the 5X5. With that kind of pedigree, it was hard to argue about the program's effectiveness.

Mehdi tried the routine and was amazed at the effect it had on him. His belly transformed into a six-pack and he gained a lot of additional muscle. "I received a lot of compliments," he recalls. "My confidence went through the roof." But it wasn't just his appearance that improved—Mehdi was stronger than ever. Not only could he beat the girls at arm wrestling, he could beat all his bros as well.

Weighing in at just about 175 pounds, Mehdi has squatted 422 pounds, bench pressed 253 pounds, and deadlifted 495 pounds—all without taking steroids!

Deciding to Drink the Kool-Aid

Pretty much everyone who hears about 5X5 believes it's too good to be true. It seems like it just doesn't make you do enough work if you really want to build muscle and increase strength. Even though I never lifted weights before, I still thought the program looked too simple to be effective when Brian was explaining it to me.

It definitely requires a leap of faith, especially during the first few weeks when you're barely breaking a sweat. But once you stop thinking about what it should look or feel like, you'll start to see that the numbers don't lie as you lift more and more weight over time. And since you only work out for forty-five minutes, three times a week, you'll have plenty of time to think about other things.

The entire workout takes a little less than two hours PER WEEK! That's half the time I spent on my simple walking routine during my McDonald's experiment. And get this—about an hour and a half of your two hours of workout time is actually spent resting.

When I first went to visit Brian at the gym, I was able to talk to some of the members and they all told me that the program works exactly as Brian said it would. It didn't matter their age or their gender, they all swore by the 5X5.

Kristy, for example, was a forty-year-old woman who started lifting weights about two years ago. "When I told them about this plan I was looking to start, they all said it was old-school weight training that would never work," she recalled to me. "That alone gave me motivation to try it!"

Even though she still thought it was a bit of a joke in the back of her mind after the first week of going through the movements, things started to change for her by the fifth week. "The increased strength I was getting was hard to believe," she told me. "I was lifting more weight than I ever had and I was doing it with ease!"

When the results started coming in, Kristy's friends were dumbfounded. They had to eat crow, because this "old-school" training program was doing everything it promised—and more.

The other stories were similarly remarkable. Phoebe, age twenty, started the 5X5 at the suggestion of her boyfriend, and when he saw how strong she was getting, he quit his gym and joined MuscleBoundUSA.

"Whether you're a man or a woman, being physically strong makes you more adaptable for life," Phoebe said to me. "It makes you less vulnerable, and when you look and feel stronger, it gives you a sense of self-confidence. My goal is not to put on muscle mass but to simply get and stay strong. It's a lifestyle change, and this program doesn't take huge amounts of time to do like many programs require."

One young man I spoke with, a twenty-two-year-old named Spencer, told me that he was never much of an athlete. "I was a skinny marshmallow," he said. "I rarely exercised and ate a lot of food filled with fat and sugar."

It sounded to me like a diet most Americans can relate to!

"When I first listened to what this 5X5 program was all about, I thought there was no way this would work," he recalled. "It seemed way too easy. Even after the first two weeks I was thinking the same thing. The workout wasn't even an effort to do. After the fifth week, however, I could feel myself getting stronger and was lifting more than I ever had. I was sold at that point, and have been doing it now for about twelve weeks and have never been stronger or more fit."

Anthony had basically the opposite story. In high school he weighed 315 pounds. He could bench 265 pounds and squat 315 pounds. However, his strength was steroid induced, and he got soft when he stopped playing sports and taking drugs.

"One day I just happened to come into the gym to see what it was all about," he told me. "At that time, I weighed 285 pounds and none of it was muscle. After hearing how the program worked, I said to myself, no way." Although skeptical, he gave it a try and achieved remarkable results. In just three months he lost more than 75 pounds. At a svelte 212, Anthony was benching 92 percent of his body weight a total of twenty-five times in a given workout. To put that in perspective, when he was in high school and on steroids, he could only bench press 84 percent of his weight a single time! Granted, he weighed a lot more back then, but still!

During our conversation I asked him what the biggest difference was between his high school days working out with steroids versus exercising naturally on the 5X5. "My mood changes back then were really big," he said. "I get much less pissed off now and have a much better disposition. I actually feel stronger now than I ever did. And now that I'm eating cleaner my body is operating much more efficiently. You really can get stronger naturally, and I tell kids all the time not to take the easy way out by trying steroids."

Levi, age nineteen, had been lifting weights since he was a high school sophomore. He spent two hours a day, three days a week, lifting weights. He got pretty strong benching a max of 190 pounds, squatting 340 pounds, and deadlifting 405 pounds, but it ate into his social life and his studies.

"I worked hard and thought that the soreness I got every day meant I was getting something out of it. Yes, I got stronger, but I never realized I wasn't giving my body enough recuperation time. Once I came across the 5X5 program my immediate thought was that this just wasn't hard enough. The first week I didn't even break a sweat. I kept with it, and after four weeks I started realizing there was something to this program as I blew by my previous personal records with ease."

James has been a serious lifter for the past seven years. His typical routine, which he did four days a week, was to go full blast for two torturous hours. He had stalled out on his strength gains—most likely from overtraining!—and decided to give the 5X5 program a try. I asked him what he thought when the 5X5 was explained to him.

"My response was, 'Are you serious?'" he told me. "I had always equated sweat and pain as part of getting strong, and in that first week not only did I not break a sweat, but I felt like I wasn't doing anything. Then at about the four-week mark things started changing. I absolutely went way over what I had ever lifted before by 40 or 50 pounds. It was then I realized that the smaller weight increases, and more rest was indeed the key to getting stronger."

Okay, so these people—all of them considerably younger than me—drank the Kool-Aid. Big deal, right? I was a middle-aged guy with no lifting experience, so maybe I was more justified in my skepticism. At any rate, I only had their opinions to go by. I really couldn't judge the program fairly until I tried it for myself and tracked my data over at least a twelve-week time frame.

I thought, "What have I got to lose?" I've never lifted weights before, but I have a good work ethic and I knew that after sticking to the parameters of the McDonald's project for six months, I could easily do this for three months.

It would be a small price to pay to turn my biological clock back a few years.

As the perfect human lab rat, I signed up to begin another grand experiment that would hopefully change my life for the better.

Learning the Basics

On the first day of training, Brian spent time trying to figure out where my starting weights should be in each of the five lifts, which I'll explain in a second.

"Why don't we just see what my maximums are in each of the five lifts?" I asked innocently.

"Absolutely not!" he said sternly. "Your body is nowhere near being able to put that kind of stress on it without hurting yourself." He told me that we'd test for my max lifts about every three weeks, but not until my body developed a stable baseline. He spent that first day teaching me the form needed to perform each exercise properly with very light weights.

The name "5X5" describes the program. You lift a specific weight five times in a row for each set, and you do five sets of each exercise. And on any given workout day, you do this "5X5" routine for three different exercises.

Here's how the routine breaks down. Note that it takes two weeks (six workouts) to do a complete cycle, and then everything repeats:

Monday

Squat	5 sets of 5 reps each
Rest	2– 2.5 min. between sets
Military Press	5 sets of 5 reps each
Rest	2–2.5 min. between sets
Dead Lift	5 sets of 5 reps each
Rest	2–2.5 min. between sets

Wednesday

Squat	5 sets of 5 reps each
Rest	2–2.5 min. between sets
Bench Press	5 sets of 5 reps each
Rest	2–2.5 min. between sets
Bent Over Row	5 sets of 5 reps each
Rest	2–2.5 min. between sets

Friday

Squat	5 sets of 5 reps each
Rest	2–2.5 min. between sets
Military Press	5 sets of 5 reps each
Rest	2–2.5 min. between sets
Dead Lift	5 sets of 5 reps each
Rest	2–2.5 min. between sets

Monday

Squat	5 sets of 5 reps each
Rest	2–2.5 min. between sets
Bench Press	5 sets of 5 reps each
Rest	2–2.5 min. between sets
Bent Over Row	5 sets of 5 reps each
Rest	2–2.5 min. between sets

Wednesday

Squat	5 sets of 5 reps each
Rest	2–2.5 min. between sets
Military Press	5 sets of 5 reps each
Rest	2–2.5 min. between sets
Dead Lift	5 sets of 5 reps each
Rest	2–2.5 min. between sets

Friday

Squat	5 sets of 5 reps each
Rest	2–2.5 min. between sets
Bench Press	5 sets of 5 reps each
Rest	2–2.5 min. between sets
Bent Over Row	5 sets of 5 reps each
Rest	2–2.5 min. between sets

As you can see, the squat is the one exercise you do during every workout. It's such a powerful exercise! Not only does it work your legs, it strengthens your core and even your upper body. When your strength improves and you start lifting heavier weights while still keeping perfect form, your heart rate goes up and you feel pretty winded after just five repetitions. Your whole body gets into the act when you're doing squats, and that's why they are so central to this program.

The other four exercises are also compound movement exercises, and all five together give your body total overall strength. By utilizing compound movements you incorporate multiple muscle groups at the same time, so it's much more efficient than doing lots of isolation exercises for individual body parts.

Brian helped me establish my starting points for each exercise based on some observation of my form and his experience working with people from all backgrounds. He was definitely conservative with me, so some of the starting points were actually lower than what I could have handled. That's why we raised some of the weights more than usual later in the program.

John Cisna—5X5 Program Starting Weights

Week	Squat	Bench Press	Overhead Press	Deadlift	Bent Row
1	115	95	65	135	100

The 5x5 Exercises

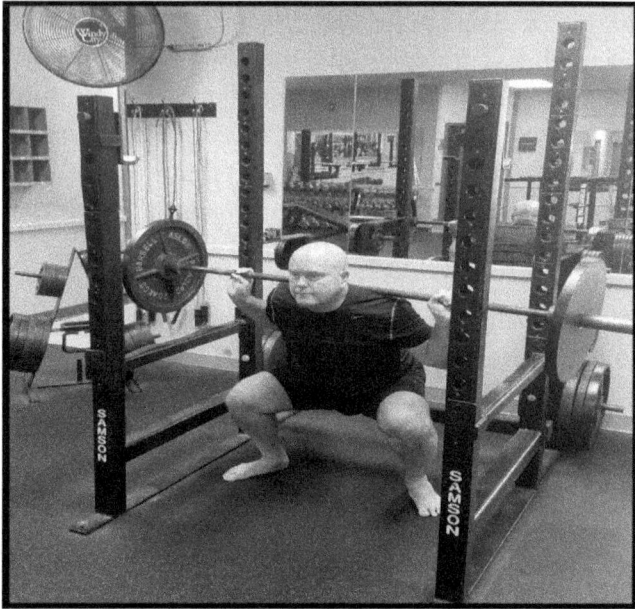

Squat – Starting Position

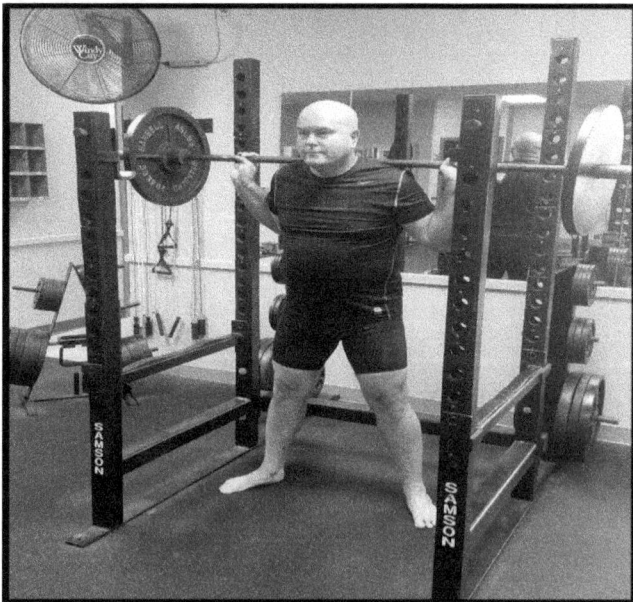

Squat – End Position

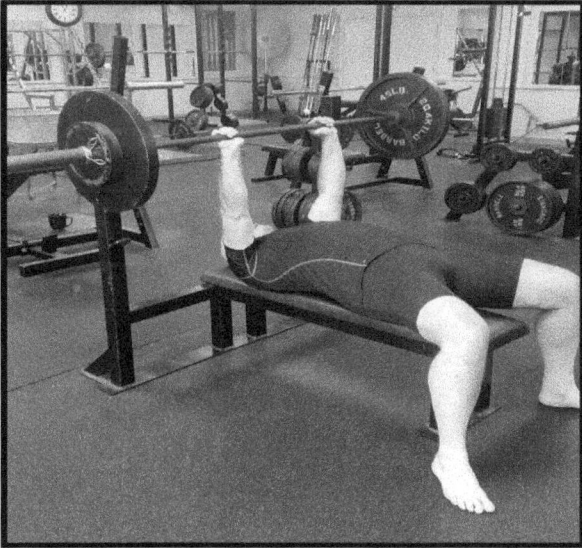

Bench Press

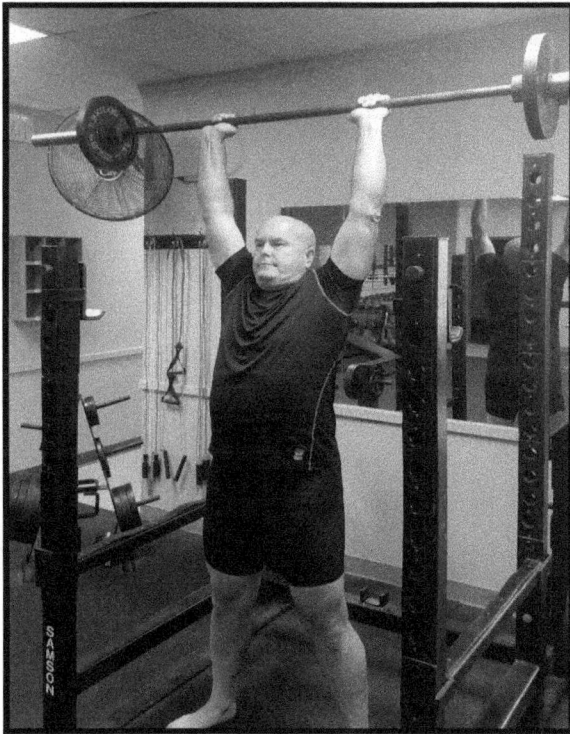

Overhead Press

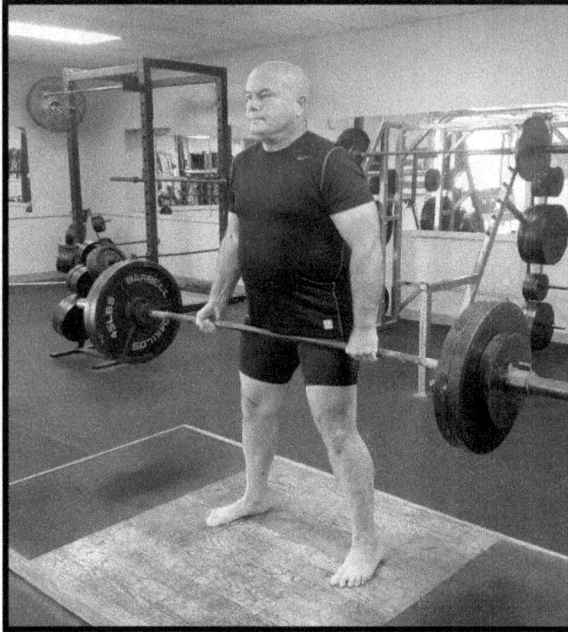

Deadlift

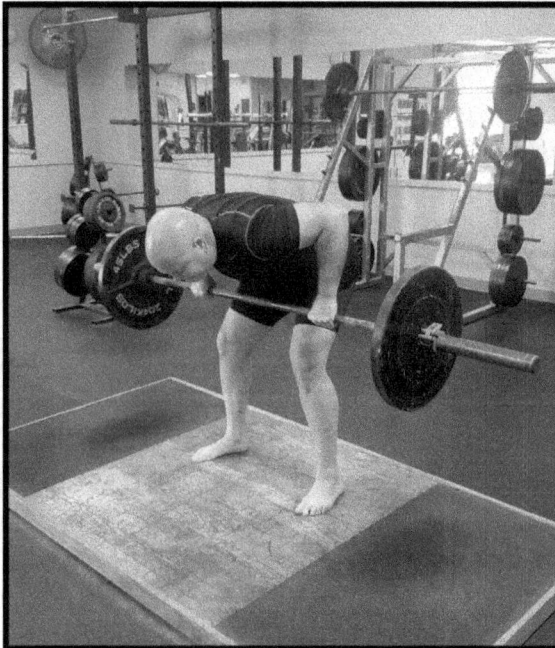

Bent Row

A Sore Lifter

Any athlete will tell you that the toughest part of starting up a new exercise routine isn't the first day, but the day after. That's when Mr. Lactic Acid comes by to pay you a little visit, and he is a most unwelcome guest indeed.   Lactic acid is a byproduct of the anaerobic reaction that occurs when muscle fibers are stressed. And when lactic acid builds up in your tissue, it causes the kind of muscle soreness that can make it next to impossible to get up in the morning and move through your day if you're not used to training.

In a nutshell, your body likes to use oxygen to help generate the energy it needs. However, sometimes when you do something strenuous, your body needs more energy than the available oxygen can supply. That's when your body uses glucose to pick up the slack. This generates lactate, which builds up in your muscles and increases their acidic level. Gentle movement for a few days after a strenuous workout is what works the lactic acid out of your system and removes the soreness.

On my first day of training, I did five sets of squats with 115 pounds on my shoulders. This type of training was foreign to my quadriceps, so when I went in for my appointment with the commode the next morning, my legs buckled and I sat down with a terrible crash.

"Are you okay?" yelled my wife from the bedroom.

I was laughing so hard I had tears in my eyes, and I could barely lift myself off the toilet. It would have been a perfect Candid Camera moment!

A Recovering Weightlifter

In his forty-five years of weightlifting, my trainer Brian has come to learn that the biggest mistake most people make is not giving themselves enough recovery time between workouts. As I found after just one day of training for forty-five minutes, lifting weights is one of the most stressful activities you can put your body

John Cisna

through. We know what it does to your muscles, and scientists are just beginning to understand that it stresses your nerves as well.

So if you don't give your body the chance to rest and repair itself, your progress will eventually stall and your risk of injury will go way up. There's a reason Major League pitchers need four days of rest before they can go out and play again. So it is also with weight training. You actually become stronger during your rest periods. When you lift properly, you create little micro-tears in your muscle fibers, so by the time you're finished training you're a bit weaker than you were when you started your workout. The process your body goes through to heal these tears and prepare your muscles for lifting more weight is what builds bigger muscles and, perhaps more importantly, protects you from injury.

If you train harder than you can recover, you're eventually going to experience the nasty symptoms of overtraining. Unlike being an overachiever, this is not a good thing. If you do too much work in the gym without enough rest, then your workouts will stagnate, you might injure yourself and get sidelined for weeks or months, your strength and energy will actually decrease, and you may even lose the motivation you had to get fit and healthy.

When you start the 5X5 program, you're not even going to feel like you're working hard enough. You probably won't even be sore the next day, and you'll be tempted to pile on the weight to make it more difficult. That will only impede your progress, so resist the temptation! Soon enough, you'll be showing off your strength, so be patient and do it when it counts.

Slow and steady wins the race when it comes to the 5X5. Each week you're only going to add five pounds to each exercise. It doesn't seem like much, but at the end of twelve weeks—just three months—you'll be lifting sixty more pounds in each exercise than when you started. I couldn't even bench 60 pounds when I began the program, so I doubled the amount of weight I was doing in that exercise in a single season. At the time of this writing, I'm benching an impressive 175 pounds during my workouts and my maximum is 235.

Since you're increasing the weight so gradually, the lifts pretty much always seem easy to do. At some point, however, you'll reach your body's natural limits and simply won't be able to complete all twenty-five repetitions of a given exercise. At that point, it's time to dial back the weight a bit and slowly go at it again, always striving to test your genetic limits.

The things that are totally out of your control, like the length and density of your bones and the shape and composition of your muscle tissue, are the things that really determine how strong you can be.

Most people on the 5X5 program start to realize their new strength by the third or fourth week of the program. And it's pretty remarkable when you can look in the mirror and say, "Wow! I'm getting stronger naturally!"

Let the Gains Begin

Despite my initial soreness, I followed Brian's program of three work days and four rest days a week pretty religiously. I paid attention to my form and I started feeling stronger after only a couple of weeks. We even went up in weight more quickly in the squat and the deadlift because I was handling the weights so well. Like I mentioned earlier, my start weights in some exercises were lower than they could have been, so I could work on getting the proper form down.

At the end of the third week I was feeling particularly good and asked Brian if we could test my deadlift just to see where I was. This was one of my stronger lifts and I wanted to see for giggles and snorts the maximum I could lift one time. Brian kind of smiled and told me I was not going to believe what I could do. With his background, he seemed like he was able to sense the kind of strength I had when I didn't have a clue about what I could or couldn't handle.

We were working with 165 pounds during my normal deadlift sets that particular week, and I told him it would be great if I could lift 240 pounds.

He smiled at me and started putting weights on the bar without telling me how much it was. I'd do a single lift, and if it felt good, he'd add more weight. We repeated the process until we got to a point where he said this was as far as he'd let me go. I got psyched up and pulled with all I had, and even though it felt very heavy, it went up without much of a problem.

He smiled again and told me the shocking news—I had just deadlifted 300 pounds!

Here I was almost fifty-eight years old, without any history of weight training, and I was lifting what most men my age couldn't even come close to after just three weeks of training. I was pumped!

I remembered the adrenalin rush I got when, halfway through my McDonald's project, my blood work came back for the first time and proved that I was getting healthier. I now got that same rush just seeing how my strength was improving in just a short amount of time.

My strength gains continued to be phenomenal, and I actually ENJOYED going to the gym at the start of each new week to see if I could tackle the new weights. It was a great feedback loop to keep progressing and gaining the kind of confidence that comes from continuous improvement. I knew that one day I'd plateau, but the constant gains over the first weeks and months really made me feel good!

Just take a look at my progress charts and you'll see that the numbers don't lie. By the sixth week, I was squatting with 205 pounds. My deadlift was up to 185 pounds. My bench was a respectable 130, my bent row was 135, and even my weakest lift, the overhead press, went up by 50 percent from the day I started.

At the end of my eighth week, we decided to test my maximums again on my best exercises, the squat and the deadlift. Starting with the squat, I watched Brian load up three forty-five-pound plates on each side of the bar, which also weighed 45 pounds. It looked like only a monster could move it, but I knew that Brian wouldn't put on an amount of weight that would hurt me. I trusted him completely at this point!

To my amazement, I was able to do a full squat with 315 pounds with no leg wraps and no belt. What was even more amazing is that I knew I could do even more! Not bad for a guy who's been eligible for an AARP card for nearly a decade!

Two days later came the deadlift. I warmed up —WARMED UP!—with 185 pounds, then did some reps at 225. Once I felt loose we put on 265 pounds, then 315, then 365! It went up without a problem. I told Brian I had one more in me, so he added twenty more pounds and I stepped up to the bar. When I started lifting it, I could feel every bit of the 385 pounds, but slowly the bar went up and I locked it in.

Just five weeks earlier my maximum deadlift was 300 pounds, and I just shattered that record by almost 33 percent! When I started this training, I wanted to squat 300 pounds and deadlift 400 pounds by the end of one year! Two days earlier I had already passed the first goal with the squat, and here I was just 15 pounds shy of my annual deadlift goal after just eight weeks.

I posted videos of my squat and deadlift records on my Facebook page, and Brian posted my deadlift on his. The videos attracted a lot of comments. They were mostly from amazed friends and family members, but a lot of "expert" weightlifters came out of the woodwork to say that my form was terrible and that I'd really hurt myself if I wasn't careful.

I learned from my McDonald's experiment that critics always go after people who do dare to something out of the ordinary. I've learned not to take it personally, but part of me wanted so badly to say to these people, "Don't you find it at least a little bit amazing that a fifty-eight-year-old man can lift 385 pounds off the ground?" How much better off would our society be if more people pushed the limits of their physical and mental faculties by trying to improve themselves?

I'm all for constructive criticism, but it's something else to be downright mean or accuse me of not really lifting the weight because I didn't do it right.

One of the reasons Brian captures personal record attempts on video is so we can review the lifts. As a former coach, I can attest to the fact that when you try to teach an athlete a different way of doing something, it can go fine on the practice field but fall apart in a real, competitive situation. That's exactly what happened to me in these heavy lifts. I went back to my old habits and proper form went right out the window.

John Cisna

Knowing that there was lots of room for improvement in my form, I decided to make that the focus of my workouts from then on. We backed my squat down to 155 pounds and lowered my bench to 115 pounds. The overhead press was my weakest lift and I moved that back from 90 pounds to 75 pounds. Although I felt very strong in the bent over row, I also moved that from 140 pounds back to 105 pounds so I could work on my back alignment. And finally, I moved the deadlift from 200 pounds back to 175 pounds.

When you back down, or reset, it gives you a chance to really work on form so heavier weights won't become a problem that results in an injury. It's kind of like a baseball swing in that once you see the results of hitting it hard and getting the *"feeling,"* then it becomes second nature. So I found it to be true with lifting weights. Remember what I mentioned earlier in the book, that the key is patience! There is absolutely nothing wrong with resetting your weights over and over in an attempt to get better form. All that does is prepare your body for weight increases while minimizing the chance of injury. If you go into this program with no timeline and no goal other than to get strong and healthy, then time is on your side.

While testing my maximums is fun every now and then, I'm not looking to break any geriatric records for weightlifting, and I'm certainly not in any kind of a race. I simply want to get as strong and as healthy as I possibly can, and I'm going to let my body lead the way. Light workouts have dramatically increased my strength, and they'll continue to do so until I've reached my natural physiological and mental limits.

Leave Your Ego at the Door

Shortly after I posted my lifting videos on Facebook, I got another sign from God that a little humility might do me some good. From 2001 through 2004, my wife Kim and I lived in Scottsdale, Arizona, with our three daughters. Our next-door neighbors were Dr. Henry Sanel, his wife, Anne Mie, and their daughter, Celine. Our two families became pretty close in those four years, and we always make a point to get together with Henry and Anne Mie whenever we're back in the great American Southwest.

Kim and I were in the desert after I'd been on the 5X5 program for a while, and we happily accepted a dinner invitation at the Sanel residence. During the course of the dinner, we talked about what we were all up to, and when it was my turn I started telling them about my new plant-based diet (more on that later) and weightlifting lifestyle.

Henry has always taken very good care of himself and plays tennis a couple times a week. He's in very good shape for a guy in his late sixties and is very conscientious about what he eats. He was very happy to hear about my new plant-based food plan. As I described the foods I was eating in great detail, he kept nodding his approval of everything on the menu!

When I started talking about the 5X5 program, however, he had a major attitude adjustment. When I told him that after just eight weeks I could squat 315 pounds and deadlift 385 pounds, he looked very concerned as only a medical doctor can.

"Do you have some concerns about this?" my wife asked.

Henry and his wife are pain management physicians. He treats patients who have chronic pain, and he has extensive experience with middle-aged and older patients.

"As people get older, we all get differing levels of increased disc herniation in our spines," he said. "This is part of the normal process of aging. Virtually everyone over forty has disc herniations, and they don't typically cause pain in most people. When you add increased levels of stress to these compromised discs by lifting very heavy weight, however, you can greatly increase these herniations."

He went on to say that "discs subjected to an inordinate amount of stress may become permanently damaged, causing chronic pain for the rest of a person's life. Even if recovery is possible, when discs are damaged in middle-aged and older people, the recovery time may take months or even years. In addition to this, lifting very heavy weight can cause muscles and tendons to tear in older people. Humans, in general, were simply not designed to lift this kind of heavy weight, much less people our age."

Henry's lecture was kind of heavy, so we moved onto a few lighter topics while we finished our dinner. After the meal was over, Henry asked if I wanted to walk the dogs with him.

"Sure," I said.

During our walk, I brought up our dinner conversation again because my conscience was getting the better of me. I asked him for more thoughts on this weight program I was on and he gave me some great insights.

"Is your goal to get healthier and stronger and maintain this level of conditioning, or is your goal to lift the most amount of weight possible?" he asked.

Before I could even start to answer, he went on to say, "If your goal is what I think it is, then is the risk of chronic injury worth it for you to jeopardize your strength program for one moment of lifting a huge amount of weight?"

He was very professional and eloquent in basically saying, "Leave your incredible ego at the door!"

OMG! Was he right? Were my competitiveness, cockiness, and ego getting in the way of my REAL goals?

I've always respected Henry's opinions—as both a doctor and a friend—and I told him that I'd take his concerns to heart when I went back to Iowa and started lifting again.

At this point it suddenly occurred to me I may never lift more than the 315 pounds I squatted and the 385 pounds I pulled off the floor in the deadlift. I had to think seriously if I'd be willing to risk my long-term goals for a few short minutes of bragging rights.

When I got back I discussed this conversation with Brian. He agreed fully with Henry, except to say that developing muscle strength gradually over time greatly reduces the chance of herniating disks or getting any other injury. Bringing it back to baseball again, you can't just go out and throw a ball 90 mph without first training your arm to do so. Without the proper training, a pitcher could do major damage trying to do too much too soon.

The chart on the following page shows my progress during my first twelve weeks in the 5X5 program. You'll notice that we made some weight adjustments early on in order to find the right amount of weight for each exercise. You want to put in some effort, but it shouldn't feel too stressful to complete all twenty-five repetitions of each exercise.

Getting Stronger Every Day

Week	Squat	Bench Press	Overhead Press	Deadlift	Bent Row
1	115	95	65	135	100
2	120	105	70	140	105
3	155	120	75	165	115
4	175	125	80	175	120
5	180	130	85	180	125
6	205	135	90	185	130
7	205	110*	75*	190	135
8	210	115	75	195	110*
9	180*	120	80	200	115
10	185	125	80	205	120
11	190	130	85	210	125
12	195	135	85	215	130
*Reset					

John Cisna

An asterisk represents a point where I had to "reset" to a lower weight. Once it gets difficult to do five reps five times with a certain weight, it means you need to back off, or reset, and build back up so that the weight is more manageable when you get to it again down the road. When your body maxes out at some point, your workouts will become cap and reset over and over again.

Is Variety the Spice of Life?

The beauty behind the 5X5 program is that after the first twelve weeks—once you've built a solid foundation of overall strength—you can deviate, if you choose, to reach any new goals you may have, such as shaping your physique and refining its appearance.

In my case, I had wanted to focus on getting my midsection a little tighter by losing more fat. This required training that was more cardiovascular in nature, which means getting your heart rate up for sustained periods of time.

To reach this goal, Brian changed my weightlifting program to a 4X10 protocol. I still did the same five exercises, but instead of doing five sets of five repetitions of each movement on a given day, I did four sets of ten repetitions. In other words, I did forty total repetitions of each exercise instead of twenty-five.

To make this possible and optimally effective, I used less weight and cut my rest time between sets to about fifteen seconds to keep my heart rate elevated for the duration of the workout. Because I was moving faster, each workout only took about fifteen minutes instead of the usual forty-five.

This protocol won't increase your strength like the original program does, but it can increase your endurance and help you burn fat quicker.

I didn't like this program nearly as well, and after just two weeks I punted it. I was one tired old man after those short workouts! I was sweating considerably, breathing heavily, and was so taxed physically that my hands would shake uncontrollably for about ten minutes. THAT was the type of workout I was trying to avoid, so it was back to the 5X5 program that I continue to this day.

I might take on the intensity of the 4X10 again if I really get bothered by my midsection, but for now I'm willing to live with my body the way it is to avoid putting myself through that kind of torture.

I know I can always add moderate exercise, like walking, to my program and adjust the amount of calories I consume in order to burn more fat. And, as you'll read later, I've been experimenting with apple cider vinegar, which has turned out to be a terrific fat burner for me.

We're all on our individual journeys through life, and for me it's important to do three things:

1. Accept the limits of my unique physiology
2. Only do things that I'm comfortable doing
3. **Keep experimenting to make gradual improvements**

The older I get, the more I realize that this is, for me at least, the right formula for success.

$25/Month for the Testosterone of a 25-Year-Old

If there's one single factor in becoming physically strong and healthy, for men especially, it's the level of testosterone running through your body. Testosterone is the basic fundamental building block of muscle development.

As I alluded to earlier, testosterone levels peak in our twenties and start to decline at the rate of one to two percent each year beginning around age thirty. That means that a man of my age, fifty-eight, will have less than 50 percent of the testosterone he had in his prime.

While low testosterone does affect the libido, it has even more sinister effects on the body. "Low T" contributes to obesity and fatigue, and it can accelerate type 2 diabetes, cardiovascular disease, and prostate cancer.

John Cisna

Al Sears, America's leading anti-aging doctor, is a big proponent of keeping testosterone levels high. According to Dr. Sears, research from all over the world shows that the more testosterone you have, the less chance you'll die—of ANY cause!

Writing in "What Men Really Need to Boost Testosterone," an article you can find on alsearsmd.com, Dr. Sears referenced six startling studies that all highlight the benefits of high testosterone levels. "It doesn't matter how old you are, your body fat, cholesterol, blood pressure, or what your blood sugar measurements are," he asserted. "In all the studies, testosterone was the biggest indicator of longer lifespan."

Here's a quick overview of the studies he was referring to:

- *In 2010, researchers found that men with heart disease are twice as likely to die if they also have low testosterone levels.*
- *A 2009 study of men with diabetes showed that those with the lowest T levels were twice as likely to die— not just from diabetes but for any reason.*
- *A European study showed that low testosterone led to a 41 percent greater chance of dying from any cause.*
- *The University of California looked at 794 men over a time period of about 12 years. They found that men with low testosterone were 40 percent more likely to die than those with higher levels.*
- *A study of older men in Seattle, published by the Journal of the American Geriatrics Society, found that those with low testosterone were 28 times more likely to die.*
- *And in a study on military veterans, low testosterone upped the risk of death by 88 percent.* For citations of all these studies, go to Dr. Sears's article at: alsearsmd.com/2011/04/a-new-look-at-what-men-really-need/ and scroll down to the footnotes.

You can do all the research you want, but I'm pretty sure all you need to know is that the testosterone so crucial to saving lives is called free testosterone. It's called that because there are no proteins attached to it. It is literally free to enter cells and activate receptors to make men more virile. You want as much free testosterone as you can get, but you may be surprised that it makes up only about two to three percent of your total testosterone.

The other two kinds of testosterone, which make up the vast majority of the testosterone in our bodies, are attached to proteins and are biologically inactive. They really don't matter too much for our purposes here, although doctors sometimes lump albumin-bound testosterone (ABT) in with free testosterone when they check for testosterone levels.

I believe it's the free testosterone that's the important stuff. Most doctors will tell you that free T is the determining factor in how much muscle mass you can create, so that's really the major thing you should test for if you're interested in getting your testosterone levels checked.

The good news is that diet and exercise have been shown to have an impact on the amount of free testosterone we have. One of the most intriguing studies that I found came out of Iran, which basically recommends that guys like us eat a lot of onions. Onions are high in antioxidants, which have been shown to increase testosterone levels. In this particular study, rats who got a gram of onion juice (per kilogram of body weight) injected directly into their stomachs saw a 300 percent increase in testosterone after twenty days.

Another group of rats was fed a casein diet, and half of them were also given garlic powder. After twenty-eight days, you guessed it—the garlic-gobbling rats had higher testosterone levels.

Now I don't know if these studies apply to humans, but I'm not taking any chances. I eat garlic and onions a lot more than I used to!

Going to the gym is definitely helping to boost my testosterone levels, and the twenty-five dollars a month I pay for my membership is half the price of some of the popular testosterone supplements on the market today. And it's a whole lot less expensive than the injections and creams that many doctors prescribe.

Brian talks a lot about getting the steroid effect from the right combination of diet and exercise, and he should know because he's walked both sides of the steroid line and knows how much better it is to boost testosterone naturally.

Brian started lifting weights at age ten, but using steroids never occurred to him until he won a Mr. Teen Iowa contest at age nineteen.

"The rush I got from winning was addictive, and I started using steroids in the quest to become a national competitor," Brian recalls. He won many competitions between 1978 and 1983, standing five feet seven inches and weighing 240 pounds of solid muscle. "I was big and I was ripped," he says.

Anabolic steroids, or anabolic-androgenic steroids (AAS), are the synthetic (made in a lab) derivatives of the naturally produced hormone testosterone. They promote the growth of muscle (anabolic effect) and the typical male characteristics of puberty (androgenic effect).

When we lift weights heavier than what we're used to, we create tiny micro-tears in muscle fibers. The body's natural repair process repairs these tears and then overcompensates by adding bigger cells to build a stronger fiber—this is called muscular hypertrophy. Over time, this repeated process of teardown and rebuild can result in muscle growth. Natural testosterone is the body's main ingredient for this process, and adding steroids accelerates the process.

Once ingested, an AAS travels through the blood stream to the muscle tissue. It is drawn into the muscle cell's receiving dock, called an androgen receptor. Once delivered to the muscle cell, the steroid can interact with the cell's DNA and stimulate the protein synthesis process that promotes cell growth.

Different variants and amounts of AAS can cause different reactions, producing either massive bodybuilding physiques or more toned athletic muscles. Athletes experiment with different combinations (called stacking) and regimens (pyramiding) in an attempt to fine-tune the final results.

The bodybuilding lifestyle consumed Brian, but one day his wife gave him an ultimatum—which was it going to be, bodybuilding or your family? Brian gave up bodybuilding and chose his wife and kids.

As he cycled off steroids through the course of a year, he dropped 60 pounds and lost a significant amount of strength, size, and definition. "I struggled with just being a normal guy even though I was still very muscular."

It wasn't until 2012—after years of bad eating, drinking, and generally unhealthy living—that he decided to focus on his health and get more disciplined in his lifestyle.

"At this time in my life I was fairly strong and fit looking, but I really didn't feel that great," Brian told me. "So I prayed for guidance and began to study food and nutrition night and day. One day I thought, what would happen if a person combined the best food program with the best workout program? After much research I combined the 5X5 strength program with a modified plant-based food regimen. Over the course of two years I found the 'steroid effect' I was looking for."

What Brian means by the steroid effect is the combination of diet and exercise that boosts testosterone and creates a stronger, more muscular, youthful body without the harmful side effects.

When he used steroids in the 1970s and early 1980s, Brian could train a lot harder and recover a lot faster, which meant more gains in a shorter period of time. His body functioned better as well—he got more sleep and had more energy, and his libido was through the roof.

The initial results people get from using steroids can be extremely gratifying, especially in this day and age of aesthetics and the importance of performance. But the big problem with steroids is that they have long-term negative side effects. And since they can be addictive, the side effects can be incredibly severe in people who abuse steroids. Brian knew lots of guys who took more and more steroids in their quest to get bigger and stronger, sometimes never cycling off like you're supposed to. Many of his peers passed away early in life, and those who survived their steroid abuse are all dealing with serious health issues.

The National Institute on Drug Abuse lays out the harsh reality:

> Steroid abuse disrupts the normal production of hormones in the body, causing both reversible and irreversible changes. Changes that can be reversed include reduced

sperm production and shrinking of the testicles (testicular atrophy). Irreversible changes include male-pattern baldness and breast development (gynecomastia).... Steroid abuse has been associated with cardiovascular diseases (CVD), including heart attacks and strokes, even in athletes younger than 30. Steroids contribute to the development of CVD, partly by changing the levels of lipoproteins that carry cholesterol in the blood. Steroids, particularly oral steroids, increase the level of low-density lipoprotein (LDL) and decrease the level of high-density lipoprotein (HDL). High LDL and low HDL levels increase the risk of atherosclerosis, a condition in which fatty substances are deposited inside arteries and disrupt blood flow. If blood is prevented from reaching the heart, the result can be a heart attack. If blood is prevented from reaching the brain, the result can be a stroke.

Most men today don't experience the healthful "steroid effect" because they eat poorly, don't exercise properly, don't get enough sunlight, and get exposed to harmful chemicals. Declining testosterone levels have been the trend for decades.

While testosterone replacement is becoming very popular, it's just an artificial shortcut with its own risk factors. Doctors are very quick to prescribe testosterone injections and creams, while discounting the effects of a better diet and exercise. Brian has seen many of his gym members increase their testosterone levels just by following his program, and they get the added benefit of using their bodies for the physical activity they were designed to perform. It feels good to move!

Like Brian, I believe that the steroid effect is possible for everyone. Brian tells me that when he put his program together, it was like rolling the clock back twenty or thirty years.

"If you give your body what it needs—good food, exercise, sunlight, and reduced chemical exposure—it will continue to dumbfound you by getting stronger and healthier," Brian said to me. "People need to stop listening to the lies that suggest that they might be over the hill or that they could never look a certain way or accomplish a certain thing. Listen, 'Get Muscle—Age Don't Matter' is what we truly believe is the key to good health."

Chapter Five

A Plant-Based Diet
You Can Sink Your Teeth Into

I ate like a pig the other day. And for five months I haven't counted a single calorie. But the amazing thing is—I feel a lot better now than I have for the past twenty years.

When I hit forty, my friends started calling me Snackbar. I reveled in all the food groups—particularly meat, dairy, and bread—and I wore the badge of omnivore with great pride. I was a definite steak-and-potatoes man, and there'd be hell to pay if someone dared to scrimp on the butter and sour cream. Weighing in at 280 for most of my adult life wasn't a liability, it was an ACHIEVEMENT!

Sugar was also a favorite of mine like it is for so many other red-blooded Americans. I got a big jolt of it every morning with a large bowl of Frosted Mini-Wheats, and I made sure to follow that up throughout the day with various sodas, candy bars, peanut butter and jelly sandwiches, handfuls of caramel corn, ice cream sundaes, Twinkies, and much more.

I had one rule when it came to food: If it tasted good, I'd eat a lot of it! Frankly, I never met a calorie I didn't like.

I never really thought much about what I was eating, or the impact it might be having on my health, until the days of my McDonald's experiment. Before then, I never monitored my food intake or cared a whit about what nutrients I was ingesting, let alone in what proportions.

All that changed for me when students in my sophomore biology class started telling me what I could eat at McDonald's each day based on an allotment of approximately two thousand calories.

When I started the McDonald's project, I began to see that the amount of food I put into my body had a dramatic impact on my physical appearance. And as my blood work came back from the lab every forty-five days, I became aware of food-related changes that weren't visible to the naked eye. On my McDonald's diet, I started to see the positive impact that nutrition could have on my overall health.

I took this a step further when I met Brian Gaumer. When he put me on the 5X5 strength program, he also put me on a plant-based food plan that was one hundred and eighty degrees out of phase from anything I've ever experienced with food. Before then, the only plant-based foods I ate were potatoes, burger condiments, and the occasional pizza topping. I'm not a vegetarian today, but I eat a ton more fruits and vegetables than ever and I feel a whole lot better because of it.

I won't lie to you. The thought of a big, juicy, marbled rib eye with a baked potato and a few slices of garlic bread still makes my mouth water. But I'm less likely to eat a meal like that because I'm well aware how important it is to follow a healthier food plan.

In fact, I now know that the better you eat when you're on an exercise routine, the more you'll benefit from that routine. When I taught young players how to hit a baseball, I'd constantly say to them, "Force equals mass times acceleration." I was a broken record, but I had to drum the idea into their young heads that the only things that mattered when it came to becoming a real slugger was how much mass your arms and bat had, along with how fast you could accelerate the swing.

It's the same with your overall health. If you maximize your training routine and your menu, then you maximize your health. I hate to make it sound so simple, but IT REALLY IS THAT SIMPLE!

The Protein Myth

When I first met Brian Gaumer, I got an image in the back of my mind of a Tyrannosaurus rex. I imagined him driving along country roads at night picking up wild animals to satisfy his monstrous need for protein. How else could he maintain his incredible muscle mass?

Needless to say, I was shocked to find out that the basic building blocks of his diet were plants.

I politely listened when he extolled the virtues of vegetables, although I really thought he was giving me the business. But then he said something that intrigued me: "We all have to eat, so doesn't it makes sense to find food that supplies you with the most amount of nutrients possible with the fewest number of calories?"

At that point, a light bulb went off in my head. He was telling me the same thing I had been trying to tell the world about McDonald's—that we get to control our own food choices! Why couldn't I choose to eat in a way that made me healthier and stronger?

Brian told me that foods lose important nutrients when they're processed. And because processed foods are lacking in nutrients, we have to eat more of them to get what our body needs. By eating more processed foods we might get all our nutrients, but we also get unwanted sodium, sugar, preservatives, chemicals, food coloring, and extra calories that we don't have any real use for. What we can't get rid of we store as fat, and that's not doing us any good, either.

Brian told me that I could eat whatever I wanted, as much as I wanted, as long as the food was a grown-from-the-ground vegetable in its virgin state. I definitely had mixed emotions about this. I liked the all-you-can-eat part, but I wasn't so sure about the vegetable thing. He saw the look of panic on my face at the mention of the word vegetable, and asked me to watch a movie on Netflix called *Forks Over Knives*.

I went home that night and decided to watch the documentary with an open mind. As the story unfolded I became more and more mesmerized. The science behind the benefits of a plant-based diet and the negative impact of our current high-protein, high-sugar diet really overwhelmed me.

My favorite part of the movie was when one of the doctors advocating a plant-based diet talked about how he was criticized as being too extreme. His answer was classic: He basically explained that it was a lot more extreme to let someone eat poorly, then open up his body, take veins from his legs, and sew them into his heart!

That image hit me like a ton of bricks. Have you ever seen heart bypass surgery? The surgery involves taking a healthy section of blood vessel from another part of the body, usually the leg, to bypass part of a diseased or blocked coronary artery. This creates a new passageway for blood to flow through so the heart muscle can get the oxygen-rich blood it needs to work properly.

During bypass surgery, the doctor makes a cut along the chest, usually about twelve inches in length. The breastbone is broken open and divided in half. The heart is stopped and blood is sent through a heart-lung machine. Once the surgery is over, the heart is restarted by electrical shock and recuperation begins. No, that's not extreme at all!

According to the Texas Heart Institute, five hundred thousand heart bypass surgeries occur in the United States every year. On any given day you can expect about 1,370 of our fellow citizens in an operating room getting cut open. The sad fact is that the majority of these surgeries are the result of perfectly "normal" eating habits. The choices most of us make—high sugar, high fat, high protein, and high calories with minimal or little exercise—are currently the culturally acceptable ones!

Far from being extreme, a plant-based, whole-food diet with less animal protein is one way most of us can prevent invasive surgeries like coronary bypass operations.

As I watched *Forks Over Knives*, I was impressed by the factual information that was presented, all borne out of empirical data. The scientific correlation between healthy people and a plant-based diet around the globe was eye opening.

While I didn't necessarily agree with everything—after *Super Size Me* I've become suspicious of ALL documentaries—I did see how eating this way could make me healthier than I was currently. And if I could make it a true lifestyle change, I could increase my chances of living a longer, healthier, and fuller life.

Eating Well Is Not Dieting

Forks Over Knives made me see food from a totally new perspective. It made me feel kind of stupid in a way to be completely honest. Here I was, a college-educated man with a degree in biology and I had never really stopped to consider the importance of good nutrition and a proper diet. The film made such an impact on me that I was all in to trying this plant-based food menu.

From the beginning of the McDonald's project, all the way through today, I've spent countless hours investigating diets. Weight Watchers, Jenny Craig, South Beach, Atkins, Paleo—and even my McDonald's diet. The problem with all these diets is the connotation of that miserable word—"diet."

We all know that diet can be a noun or a verb. The primary noun definition, according to the *Oxford English Dictionary*, is "the kinds of food that a person, animal, or community habitually eats." This describes normalcy in a person's food intake.

It's when you get to the primary verb definition that things get turned upside down. According to the same dictionary, the verb diet means to "restrict oneself to small amounts or special kinds of food in order to lose weight." Unlike the noun, which describes normalcy, the verb suggests a deviation of food intake.

Since you can't lose weight forever, dieting represents a short-term fix at best. And when you restrict your food intake, a lot of negative things happen to get you to stop dieting really quickly. You feel hungry all the time. You get more irritable. And your resolve weakens whenever you see a bag of chips, forcing you to eat the whole darn thing in one sitting. Dieting is no fun!

It's also ineffective, as most of us know. So, instead of trying to diet (the verb), you should simply change your diet (the noun). What Brian's food plan does is teach you how to make a better lifestyle choice when it comes to food. Instead of being restrictive, it simply becomes your new, healthier normal.

Ingredients for Success

The food plan, just like the 5X5 exercise routine, is really simple. By eating mostly plant-based foods, you get the most nutrients possible from the fewest calories possible. You don't have to count calories.

Did that register?

YOU DON'T HAVE TO COUNT CALORIES! You can eat as much as you want, when you want, and how you want, as long as what you're eating is a vegetable grown from the ground. Food that has eyes, legs, a mom, and a dad are what you want to avoid.

As I mentioned earlier, when Brian first told me the baseline rules for this food plan, I thought it was going to be very restrictive. How in the world would I go from eating all my favorite red meats, diet pops, fruit drinks, and sugary sweets to eating rabbit food?

I had to start familiarizing myself with plant-based foods I hadn't been accustomed to. It was really amazing to find out how many plant-based foods there actually are.

It was also fascinating to learn that some plant-based foods are better than others. Take nuts, for example. Walnuts and almonds are particularly good at supplying your body with the nutrients it needs, and good old-fashioned peanuts are pretty good, too. It turns out that cashews, which happen to be my favorite kind of nut, aren't that good for you. Compared to almonds, cashews have 12 percent more calories, 33 percent more sugars, 20 percent less protein, and three times the saturated fat.

Once I started looking at the foods this plan actually allows, I was able to relax. I realized, for example, that I wouldn't go without sugar: Fruit would supply me with plenty of the sweetness I was used to. After doing some investigation, I realized I could eat a lot of great things:

Vegetables
Lettuce, onions, potatoes (red or sweet), cabbage, spinach, carrots, radishes, celery, rice (brown only), beets, pickles, cucumbers, okra, broccoli, mushrooms, garlic, peppers (all colors), pumpkin, squash, and beans of all kinds.

Fruits
Bananas, apples, pineapple, cherries, berries (all kinds), papaya, oranges, pears, avocadoes, and kiwis.

Nuts
Walnuts, almonds, and peanuts are the best.

Protein
Fish and seafood (including sardines, shrimp, scallops, tuna, and salmon), chicken, tofu, and protein powder. You also

get protein from nuts, and when you eat brown rice and beans together.

Grains
Steel-cut oatmeal.

Beverages
Water, tea, and coffee.

If you focus on those foods, you should do great. Also keep in mind that you should minimize dairy products, especially cheese and milk. Pasta and bread are also discouraged, but if you do eat them, make sure they're made with whole grains only.

Sugar Ain't So Sweet

The most important thing to avoid is processed sugar and chemical sweeteners. That pretty much means no candy, sweetened cereal, cookies, juices, soda pop, and anything else containing added sugars and sweeteners. Sugar is a killer, but we keep piling it on our plates.

An interesting fact about sugar is that it's never listed in the nutrition facts label that tells you the percentage of nutrients in a serving compared to a daily calorie allowance. You'll see percentages for total carbohydrate and dietary fiber, but not for sugar.

Check it out right now. Go to your cupboard and pull down any item. See if it tells you the sugar percent of one serving of that item for the daily recommended allowance. Since it won't, I'll show you how to do the calculation yourself.

For most people, roughly no more than 10 percent of your calorie intake should be sugar. So if you consume 2,000 calories a day, no more than 200 calories should come from sugar. Each gram of sugar contains four calories, and if you divide 200 by four you get 50 grams of sugar per day.

To put this in perspective, one little can of soda contains 35 grams of sugar and a Snickers contains 30 grams of sugar. Just eating those two things puts you over your recommended daily sugar allowance by 30 percent!

John Cisna

It's obvious to me that putting the sugar percentage on our food labels would alarm people, because the percentage would be so high. Go back and look at that package that has the percentages of all the nutrients. Many of the nutrients are in the single digits for one serving. If you listed the sugar percentage, it would stick out like a sore thumb as the one ingredient that can exceed the recommended daily allowance faster than any other.

But that's not the only way we're enabling sugar use in this country. Have you seen the TV commercial that advertises toothpaste that helps keep the sugar from affecting the enamel on your teeth? The mother in the commercial basically mentions that now when her kids eat sugar, their teeth are protected. ARE YOU KIDDING ME? How about a commercial that says, "Now that my kids DON'T eat added sugar they're healthier and their teeth aren't falling out"? As silly as that sounds, instead of addressing the issue causing tooth decay, we create a fix that continues to allow overconsumption of added sugar among our youth.

Jason Wachob, the founder and CEO of Mindbodygreen, stated that the average American consumes 756 grams of sugar per day, or fifteen times what they should be eating. That's an 8,400 percent increase in the consumption of sugar!

Those grams add up to massive quantities of sugar. Mr. Wachob does the translation for us, saying that the average American eats 131 pounds of sugar a year, including 53 gallons of soda. Salt is the only other nutrient over consumed in such large quantities, and added sugar alone contributes nearly 500 calories to the average American's day.

When You're Hungry, You Eat—Sort Of

My favorite part of this food program is that you get to eat when you're hungry. That's definitely a lifestyle change I can live with. And because you never feel deprived, you really don't feel the urge to binge on high-calorie junk like you do when you're on a restricted diet. While it's highly improbable that a person could eat more vegetable calories than their body burns off, you do have to be more aware of the fruits, nuts, and grains you eat, which contain added calories.

And you've got to limit the protein. When I started the program, even though I had heard Brian and watched *Forks Over Knives*, I gave myself license to eat as much of ANYTHING on Brian's menu as I wanted, not just vegetables grown from the ground. I found out the hard way about protein when I got my first blood work done on my new food plan!

Just as I did for my McDonald's experiment, I took all my initial blood work to establish a baseline. Then I took blood on day forty-five and day ninety. Back when I was eating at McDonald's every day, every time I got blood work back I got great results, so I was excited to see what would happen now that I was REALLY eating healthy.

I actually met with my doctor the day before my results came in, bragging about what I was doing. I told him that he was going to be shocked at the results!

The next day, when I got a call from the doctor's office, I was the one who was shocked. As I started hearing the results of my blood work over the phone, I could feel the blood starting to rush from my head. I must've looked like I had just seen a ghost.

I hung up the phone and my wife asked me if I was okay. When I couldn't put a three-word sentence together, she definitely knew that something was wrong!

My cholesterol went from 259 to 261. My triglycerides went from 115 to 120. My cholesterol to HDL ratio went from 4.6 to 5.1. I immediately texted Brian and told him about the results.

He called me right away and said, "That's impossible!"

I told him it's not impossible because I had the data to prove it. He then asked me to tell him exactly what I was eating. This is where I rose to the top of the class in the stupidity rankings. I told him as long as it was grown from the ground, I was eating whatever I wanted—along with the list of protein sources he had given me as well.

"Time-out!" he said. "You can't eat whatever you want from the protein sources. Your body isn't even close to being able to eat limitless amounts of protein. That is why your numbers are so out of line!"

I felt like I had just wasted thirty days of the food plan. What an idiot I was! Brian and I decided to use my new figures as my baseline now that I really understood how the program worked. Now that the light was finally on in the attic, I would spend the next ninety days eating whatever I wanted as long as it grew from the ground.

I limited my protein intake to 6–8 ounces of salmon or tuna twice a week, plus a plant-based protein powder I'd mix into my fruit and vegetable smoothies each day.

I continued to get stronger, and was actually starting to lose a few pounds. I finally came to the end of this ninety-day period and anxiously awaited the results of this blood work. I told my wife if these results didn't come back better, she better remove all sharp objects from the kitchen or there might be a bloody mess in the house.

The results were better, but there were a couple of things I didn't like. Here are the results and how they compared with the results from the initial blood work:

	Initial	90 Days	Difference
Weight (lb.)	257.2	255.9	-1.3
Waist (in.)	49.5	45.0	-4.5
Chest (in.)	47.0	49.5	+2.5
Bicep (in.)	15.0	16.5	+1.5
Cholesterol (<200) mg/dL	261	217	-44 (-17%)
Triglycerides (<150)mg/dL	120	96	-24 (-20%)
HDL mg/dL(>40)	51	49	-2
LDL (<130) mg/dL	186	149	-37 (-20%)
Chol./HDL (<5.0)	5.1	4.4	-7
Free T levels mg/mL	45	67	+22 (+50%)

The good news is that my cholesterol dropped 17 percent and my LDL and triglycerides both dropped 20 percent. Those are pretty significant improvements in just ninety days.

The best news for me was that my testosterone levels jumped almost 50 percent, putting me well into the normal range. This will enable me to continue to get stronger—and stay alive longer!

The bad news is that although my total cholesterol and LDL were lower, they needed to drop down farther. Although I don't have any family history of heart disease, I still want to get those two figures under what's recommended.

Part of making adjustments to food plans and exercise programs is to first understand why the statistics say what they do. First, one of the things I found with this food plan is that you have to be careful of the natural sugar found in fruits. Although fruit provides additional nutritional content than sugar alone, you still must be cognizant of the amount of sugar entering your body.

Second, I was eating a fairly good amount of sweet potatoes and brown rice almost on a daily basis. The combination of the rice, potatoes, and fruit was giving me way too many carbohydrates, which are stored as fat if the body can't use them.

I learned an important lesson. Yes, you can eat as much as you want as long as it grows from the ground and is a vegetable. Grains and fruits aren't vegetables! And potatoes? Well, I guess they're the exception that proves the rule.

There was one statistic in my blood work that I just didn't understand. Your HDL level is supposed to increase the more exercise you do. I had never exercised as much in my life and I couldn't figure out how my HDL had actually gone down. I got on the Internet to do some more investigating. And then I found it: Excess carbohydrates can have a negative effect on HDL levels.

Dr. David Perlmutter is a board-certified neurologist, Fellow of the American College of Nutrition, and a *New York Times* bestselling author of books such as *Grain Brain, The Surprising Truth About Wheat*, and *Carbs and Sugar*. He's been interviewed on many nationally syndicated television programs and has received numerous awards.

About the relationship of carbohydrates to HDL, Dr. Perlmutter writes:

> *As it turns out, diet does in fact play an important role in determining a person's HDL level. In a study appearing*

in the American Journal of Clinical Nutrition, Canadian researchers evaluated the diets of 619 Canadians of either Aboriginal, South Asian, Chinese, or European descent who had no previously diagnosed medical conditions.

The researchers were particularly interested in the amount of carbohydrate intake in comparison to HDL, and what they found was really quite profound. In comparing those whose diets were highest in carbohydrate consumption with those who favored a lower carbohydrate diet, those who ate the least amount of carbohydrates had an HDL that was, on average, 11% higher.

So this is a very interesting report in that it again validates the importance of a lower carbohydrate, higher fat diet in terms of, in this case, an important cardiovascular risk marker, HDL.

This was exciting news because I was implementing the very thing I was trying to teach my students in the McDonald's project—using deductive reasoning will lead you to better choices. Now that I identified the problems, I could address them in the days ahead by eating more colored vegetables with fewer fruits and other carbohydrates.

Even though I had lost inches around my waist and gained inches around my chest and biceps, there was still plenty of fat on the land that wasn't going away as fast as it could. I joke with Brian that this plan is actually the A-H-V program, with the letters representing how your body looks as you go through the program. You start out looking like an A, then migrate to looking like an H, and finally evolving to the classic V shape with broad shoulders and a slim waist. I was in H territory, and I needed to make adjustments in order to have any hope of getting to be a V.

My experience shows how a menu plan that seems perfect for you may require adjustments based on your unique physiology. There's a reason why there isn't one food plan that works for everyone, and why it's so important to review what you're eating periodically to try to make it better. Is my diet better now than what it was? Absolutely, but it can get better still over time if I honestly compare my eating choices to the results in my blood work, on my scale, and in my mirror.

Due to the exercise, I eventually will need more food, but in the meantime, I need to get rid of the excess weight so I can start metabolizing the food coming in more quickly and efficiently.

These Are a Few of My Favorite Foods

Once you understand what you can eat and why it's important for your overall health to keep emphasizing those particular foods, it simply becomes a matter of using your imagination to come up with combinations that taste good to you.

My favorite recipe is what I call my nine-bean soup. I take a bag of nine different beans and soak them overnight in water. (You can also use bags with six types of beans and call it your six-bean soup—just use whatever is available at your store.)

The next day I drain off the water and put the beans in a big pot with spinach leaves, mushrooms, onions, carrots, celery, and broccoli.

I add fresh water to the mix and slowly bring it to a boil. After it boils for about twenty minutes, I turn down the heat, so it simmers for another thirty minutes or so. When I reduce the heat, I also add garlic, lemon, and pepper.

Sometimes I'll add a little bit of canned tuna, cooked chicken, or shrimp to the soup for protein and extra flavor, but I won't overdo it. Whether I add protein or not, every person I've served this soup to has been amazed at how good it is. Some of my friends have even started considering a plant-based diet because of it!

It's actually been pretty fun finding new ways to cook with vegetables and create new flavors by combining different vegetables with fish and seafood.

I love to cook anyway and have always done most of the cooking in our household. I just don't barbecue anymore!

The biggest challenge for me was finding sauces and dressings without high levels of sugar. I found it very common that only two tablespoons is 8-10 grams of sugar PER SERVING, which is the makeup of most dressings.

I finally found one that had only 1 gram of sugar per serving, and it was enough to make my salads more enjoyable. If you do a little research, you'll find a dressing that you like without added sugar, and later on you'll learn why this is incredibly important.

Another great way to get your veggies is to put them in a blender along with some fruit, cold water, and ice for a veggie smoothie. This may sound gross, but the fruit adds a natural sweetness that covers up the veggie bitterness. If you're not a big vegetable fan, this is definitely the way to go.

Promise me that you'll try the recipe below. I tested it out on a friend who can't stand vegetables. I had him try it and tell me what was in it. He identified all the fruits, but didn't even believe me when I told him what vegetables he had just consumed!

John's Very Veggie Smoothie

- Broccoli
- Cabbage
- Carrots
- Strawberries
- Blueberries
- One banana

Blend all the ingredients with water and pour over ice, or blend the ice right in.

Another favorite food of mine is steel-cut oatmeal (made with the least amount of processing) with bananas or some other fruit. I make my oatmeal with a small amount of water because I like it to have the consistency of yogurt with a little bit of crunchiness.

Oatmeal is a low-glycemic carbohydrate. In layman's terms, this means that oatmeal doesn't send all the carbohydrates into your body at one time. It's kind of time-released, and since it stays with you longer, you don't get hungry again quite as quickly. Many people with diabetes eat oatmeal for that reason.

If I start my day with a bowl of oatmeal, I can go several hours before I get hungry again. When I do get hungry, I eat something else. I find myself eating more frequently each day, but since the foods I eat are packed with nutrition, each meal I have is relatively small.

The strangest thing about this food plan happened to me after about four weeks in. All of a sudden, when I went to the refrigerator and saw some cherry tomatoes, I actually thought, "Boy does that look good!"

And when I picked out a handful and ate them, they tasted as good as they looked!

I also found that virtually any foods I saw that were not on this food plan didn't tempt me anymore. It's like my taste buds have evolved from that of a high-sugar, high-red meat eater into a person who actually craved highly-nutritious, low-calorie food!

I Feel Like Crap!

Brian warned me that I might experience some weakness or even flu-like symptoms about two or three weeks into my plant-based food program. He assured me that this was simply due to my body adjusting to cleaning itself up and that it would pass after a few days.

Just like clockwork, that very thing happened going into the third week. At first, I thought that I had the flu, and then remembered what Brian had said. I got through the episode okay and still managed to get my workouts in that week, even though I wasn't able to add any weight for any of the exercises.

Going through this detoxification process really pointed out that I had been abusing my body for so many years. So in a way, it was worth going through because it helped keep me motivated.

In those early weeks, when I was adjusting to my new diet, I supplemented my food consumption with vitamins B-12, B-6, and D, which I still take to this day.

Protein Has Its Place

Finding the optimal amount of protein to eat was probably the hardest part of adopting this new food plan, at least for me. I knew I had to limit my protein intake, but I also had to make sure I was eating enough to fuel my strength program.

When I started on the 5X5 program, I only ate about 6–8 ounces of fish twice a week, or about 72–96 grams of protein total.

93

John Cisna

I found very quickly that the amount of protein I was consuming wasn't nearly enough for my body. The amount someone needs varies greatly from individual to individual, as there are several factors to take into consideration.

Most nutritionists recommend about .36 g/pound of body weight for someone with a sedentary lifestyle, but you need more if you exercise on a regular basis. Building strength and muscle mass requires more protein, and now I'm eating about 150 grams of protein each day, or .59g/pound of body weight.

The key is to go by your own physiology. I simply eat what my body tells me I need. In the early days of the program I was fatigued and not feeling strong, so I increased my protein intake and immediately started feeling better. When I eat too little protein, I start to feel lethargic and weak, and when I eat too much, I start to gain weight.

I'm not eating much red meat at all—maybe once a month I'll go hog wild and order a steak, but that's about it. Instead, for day-to-day protein consumption I eat skinless chicken breasts, tuna, salmon, and a whey protein powder.

A Few T-riffic Foods

As I mentioned earlier, I'm eating onions and garlic to keep my testosterone levels up. This sounds weird, but it's really great: At night I smash up five cloves of garlic and blend it with a banana, an orange, and some water. I drink that down and chase it with a protein shake, and I feel great in the morning!

That much garlic goes through your pores, but the good news is that there isn't a vampire within miles of my house. I did solve my onion problem, however, which made my breath smell like the east end of a horse going west. My wife could hardly be in the same room with me, which kind of defeated the purpose of trying to raise my testosterone levels. Fortunately, I found that cooking onions eliminates their odorous effects without affecting their nutritional value or testosterone-building properties.

Apple Cider Vinegar Each Day
Keeps the Doctor Away

Another thing I do on a regular basis to stay healthy is take about a tablespoon and a half of apple cider vinegar every day. People claim it makes you lose weight and removes stubborn belly fat, but what I've concluded about it is that it basically helps regulate your body's pH balance and improves the efficiency of the digestive process. It also appears to create an environment that is better for the good microbes that aid in digestion.

I've lost about ten pounds since adding this ingredient to my daily routine. If you give it a try, mix it with four ounces of water and then wash it down with another four ounces of plain water. Apple cider vinegar is very acidic, and you don't want any of that acid staying in your esophagus.

Chapter Six

Next Up—YOU!

What is healthy?

When you look up the definition of "healthy," you'll find such a hodgepodge of entries that make it impossible to find a single, all-encompassing meaning. So I ask a different question: What does healthy mean for you?

When I was doing my McDonald's project, what was healthy for me was losing weight and lowering my cholesterol. Today, my body tells me that a good weight for me, given my specific food plan, exercise program, and personal goals, is about 240 pounds.

If you watch *540 Meals*, I avoid the word healthy altogether and ask, "Is it possible for a person to become better off eating nothing but McDonald's for ninety days?" It was very easy for me to answer that question by simply saying, "I went from 280 pounds to 220 pounds, my cholesterol went from 249 to 170, my triglycerides went from 156 to 80, and my LDL went from 170 to 113 on this experiment. Do you think I'm better off?"

To date, I have yet to have someone say, "No, you were better off when you looked like a whale."

If you Google my name, you'll see countless articles written about my amazing weight loss. I have yet to see one article starting out with the incredible things that happened to the inside of me. Some articles never bother to mention it at all.

Do you ever see advertisements on weight loss programs mentioning what the food plan can do for you on the inside? No! The reality of what people see as healthy revolves around what the scale says. This is so wrong!

Let's look at where I'm at with my weight training and plant-based food plan. I'm 35 pounds heavier than I was at the end of my McDonald's project, yet my blood work is pretty comparable to what it was back then. The biggest difference is in my testosterone, which has increased by an amazing 50 percent. As I continue to work out and lose more weight, I have no doubt that my blood work will continue to improve.

When I lost all that weight eating McDonald's, I appeared to be healthy, but restricting my calories wasn't really a good thing. By eating more and training harder, I have a lot more healthy muscle mass than I did at the end of my McDonald's experiment. I made the best choices I could at McDonald's given the parameters of my experiment, but I'm making much better choices today on my new program of diet and exercise.

When you restrict calories you lose weight, but you lose it everywhere! Sure your fat mass decreases, but so does your muscle mass. When I look back at the five progressive pictures taken of me during the 180 days of my experiment, all that I now see is a smaller version of myself after each period. Structurally, I didn't change that much—my stomach shrank, but so did my arms, chest, and legs.

I now understand why, when I thought I was in such good shape, I had to take four ibuprofen tablets before and after I played golf—I lost strength in addition to all the fat! My muscles had atrophied, and I had to rely on medicine to reduce the inflammation I got when I did any physical activity. Like many people, I attributed the pain to getting old, not to just being weak.

Since I've been on my weight-training program I've only had to take ibuprofen one time—after my first workout when I almost broke the toilet bowl.

Many people will look at me and say that a six-foot tall, fifty-eight-year-old man weighing 255 pounds is not healthy. Regardless of what my blood work says, and regardless of what the amount of weight I can lift says, the scale says I'm actually obese. According to standard body mass index (BMI) tables, I'm almost 70 pounds overweight!

Scales and tables are fine, but I'm here to testify that this is the best I've EVER felt physically in my life! I'm healthier and stronger now than I was twenty-five years ago. If I'm to be labeled as unhealthy and obese, then so be it, because I'm not going to try to lose 70 pounds, become less strong, and have my testosterone drop back to my previous levels.

I know what health should be—for me—and I don't care what the scale says!

Over the past four years I've learned more about health as it relates to food than I ever did in my previous fifty-four years, and my education has been a real eye opener.

As a sugar addict, I was the unhealthiest physical specimen around, and my pre-McDonald's blood work put me just one step ahead of a heart attack. My long path to better health started with a simple experiment that put my students in a box, giving them strict parameters for proving whether or not it's possible for a person to become healthier eating nothing but fast food for ninety days.

My students were dealt a hand, dirty as it may have been, where they had to think and use deductive reasoning to put meals together that would come as close to the FDA recommended standards as possible. Were they able to get all fifteen nutrients inside those standards? No! Did they get them as close as they could with the choices they had to work with? Yes!

The results simply proved the hypothesis to be true. But Morgan Spurlock proved the opposite—that a person can become less healthy eating nothing but fast food for ninety days. How is that possible? How can both be true? That's the real question, and it just comes back to the choices people make.

In EVERY speech I made, I went out of my way to make sure people understood that my experiment didn't prove you should eat fast food. It did show what could happen to an overweight person if he used a little common sense in a fast-food restaurant. It was an experiment that should have opened up people's eyes to say, "If a person can get healthier by making the best choices possible with fast food, think of how healthy someone could get when their choices aren't limited to one venue!"

I'm confident that I've found a program that will put me in the best health possible, because now I'm focused more on the nutritional value I get from foods, how strong I am, and what health problems I'm avoiding by eliminating red meat, dairy, and sugar from my diet than I am on how much I weigh or how thin I look. And I look forward to a future in which I can remain active and stay out of the healthcare system for as long as possible.

John Cisna

Imagine if every American, especially us older ones, looked at life this way?

What if doctors didn't have to perform half a million bypass surgeries every year?

What if we could eradicate food-related diabetes?

What if we could reduce high blood pressure naturally?

What if we could take most people off prescription drugs?

What if we could end the obesity epidemic once and for all?

I could go on and on with examples, but you know that the answer to all of these questions is the same: We CAN do all these things if people follow a strength-building exercise program like the 5X5 and follow a plant-based food program.

By taking individual responsibility to improve your health, you can contribute to these lofty goals. You don't have to do what I did, but you do have to know that your path to great health is out there.

If you try my program and it works for you, that's awesome. If you decide to try another way to great health, I certainly won't take it personally.

Either way I'll be happy for you, because I have a passion inside me that I didn't have four years ago, or any time since I walked into that McDonald's in Nevada, Iowa. I developed a passion for health because I've discovered firsthand how someone can turn back the clock and live life to its fullest far longer than could otherwise be expected.

I now consider myself an advocate for healthier eating and lifestyles. Am I an expert? Absolutely not. A trailblazer? I hope so. My experiences have led me to write this book and speak to audiences across the country. If I can reach just one percent of Americans considered overweight, if I can show them the power of choice to become healthier, then I'll have made a difference in two million lives!

Hey, even if just one person changes his or her life I'll be happier than an Iowa pig in mud! Will that person be you? Will you find your own Fountain of Youth? I hope so, and I hope you'll email me at info@johncisna.net. and let me know how you did it.

Acknowledgements

First and foremost, I want to thank my lovely wife of thirty-eight years for once again having patience with my experiments and me. She has been my biggest backer and fan throughout all of this. What a wonderful lifelong partner I have in her!

When I decided to put this book together, I knew I needed a great ghostwriter. Ed Sweet is the guy! He was outstanding during my first book, and the fact that he knows me so well made him the natural choice for this one. I literally could not have done either book without him.

Brian Gaumer turned out to be one of my very closest friends throughout this journey. His passion for the program he's put together, and his religious faith, sets him up in my eyes as an absolute great role model. Ask anyone in the gym and they can tell you how much they admire his leadership. You walk the talk of the Gospel—thank you, Brian!

I also want to thank all the members of MucleboundUSA who have become like a second family to me. What an incredible environment of unrelenting support! Egos are all left at the door and everyone goes out of their way to understand each other's individual goals.

I am ever grateful to Neil Cavuto of Fox News, who wrote the foreword for both of my books. He followed the first McDonald's story intently, had me on his show three times, and is one of the most honest and gracious people I've ever met. I feel very honored and fortunate to know him.

A big thank you goes to Kevin O'Brien and Jim Baker, the McDonald's owner/operators who were willing to take a risk on my initial experiment and finance all my food. If it weren't for them, neither project would have taken place.

I am also thankful that Jeff Stratton, then president of McDonald's, took an interest in my story and put his neck on the line to make my brand ambassadorship a reality. His leadership and constant backing were a source of great comfort to me during my two and a half years with the company.

Julie Barberio, my "breath of fresh air," really made the last year and a half with McDonald's a wonderful experience. WE put together one heck of a presentation, and you helped me make a difference in thousands of lives. You're the best!

And finally, the most important person I want to thank is my Lord and Savior, Jesus Christ. He is my rock and the one who fills the void that exists without Him. The hope of His promise is what drives me every day and gives me true reason for my existence. The joy I experience in this life is solely due to Him being a part of my life. Many people may question my true intent for this book. Is it money? Is it fame? I have spoken over the years of the importance of making a difference in people's lives. In these last years, I've been witness to countless people across our country who are dealing with their addiction to food and the associated problems with overcoming that addiction. Whether you're a follower in Him or not, I believe that one day we will all stand before Him. In that day he will ask, "John, what have you done for me?"

I don't want that conversation to be a difficult one. If someone has something that truly brings joy to their lives, they want others to experience the same. So it is my hope that one day every knee shall bow and every tongue confess that Jesus Christ is Lord. I put all my worries and anxieties in His hands and ask for His continued strength to lead me through these times. My life has been blessed through Him, even in the times that I wouldn't wish on my worst enemy. I hope that someday, for those of you who've read this and haven't experienced the joy of having Him in your life, you remember this writing and accept Him. It's the greatest gift that any of us will ever receive. God bless you all.

About the Author

John Cisna was born and raised in Iowa, where he currently lives with his wife of thirty-eight years—his high school sweetheart, Kim. They have three daughters, Laura, Jamie, and Dani; a cat, Salem; and a dog, Roxie. John graduated from Iowa State University with a bachelor of science in biology and a minor in education. He taught high school science for a total of ten years and still lives to be a motivator for everyone he can. John constantly tries new things, and judges the success of each day by how well he lives up to the following motto: "Today I will be the best husband, father, and friend I can possibly be, and today I WILL make a difference."

www.ingramcontent.com/pod-product-compliance
Lightning Source LLC
Chambersburg PA
CBHW050744030426

42336CB00012B/1643